Intermitt

For Beginners to Advanced - The Effective Way to Lose Weight, Burn Fat and Heal Your Body

Introduction

Actors, actresses, models and sometimes even the flight attendants look better than me! How many times have you been caught thinking on these lines only to feel demotivated and ugly at the end of this brain numbing and depressing exercise? It is a negative thought, yes, but who are you supposed to blame for this negative thinking?

Right from the time you get out of bed you are constantly bombarded with images of handsome men who look like Greek Gods, or women in their 60's claiming to run marathons and looking like they are 16 while it is a Herculean task to walk to the washroom for you? And then you begin to think and assume that all these perfect people with perfect bodies and health must be doing something radically different from you, a secret you are not aware of and you find out that most of them chant the same mantra.

The mantra is "Breakfast is the most important meal of the day." This mantra is often accompanied by "Top 5 breakfast dishes to boost your day" or "Smoothies to drive your Monday blues away."

The other very popular mantra is to "eat six small meals in a day" which essentially translates to eating almost every waking minute as there is no other way to incorporate six meals in a day considering most adult human beings sleep for 5-6 hours every day. Another big problem with eating six small meals is not everyone is equipped with the creative skills needed to make so many meals. Too many meals also mean a lot of work, which can be demotivating prompting a person to give up on the diet entirely and move back to old ways.

If breakfast is indeed the most important meal of the day, and if you have been religiously not skipping breakfast all your life even if that means gulping down a "moss colored" liquid and yet the weighing scale does not move an inch, who is to be blamed?

Your diet or you? As human beings, most of us tend to blame ourselves because clearly if the same mantra is working out for your next-door grandmother, then you must be doing it wrong. It is this myth that I am trying to bust in the book by bringing you the concept of "Intermittent Fasting."

In this book, you will be introduced to the wonderful concept of Intermittent Fasting that will not only change your life for better but will also help you achieve the body and health of your dreams.

If you are ready to toss this book as just another piece of trash, then hold on before you follow your instincts this time!! In a world where if you cannot convince then confuse seems to be the mantra that big corporations are following, it can be frustrating to not know who is lying and who is telling the truth.

I promise that by the end of this book, you will have a good understanding of Intermittent Fasting and if followed thoroughly, you will see results that will astonish you.

Thank you once again for choosing this book; let us begin.

Chapter One
What is Intermittent Fasting??

A quick Google search will throw up hundreds of articles about the benefits of fasting, the different methods to do it followed by thousands of contradicting articles claiming how each method is wrong.

If you are someone who likes to know the "how" behind something, a little digging on the internet will tell you that most research surrounding Intermittent Fasting has been dutifully and diligently carried out on, wait for it, "RATS".

Wait, what???? Rats, out of all the species inhabiting this big planet have been used to prove the theory of Intermittent Fasting. There is a lot of incredibly promising research on Intermittent Fasting that has been done on fat rats. The results have been so amazing that scientists have decided to dedicate their entire careers to spending time with rats to find results that can help us, humble human beings lead better lives.

Fret not. Intermittent Fasting might not produce all the results, but one thing it will not do is to turn you into a RAT.

Intermittent Fasting

Intermittent fasting is a brief fast where you will be required to fast for anywhere between twelve to sixteen hours or even more during a day. It is a lifestyle modification that oscillates between periods of eating and fasting. During the fasting window, you are not supposed to consume any food. Just the thought of "not eating" is enough to make some people dizzy and fall sick.
I will tell you a little secret here. The important thing to remember here is that you already fast every day without knowing it.

You might be wondering how? Just recollect any random day in your life. The first meal of the day is called "breakfast" which is had after a gap of at least 6 hours at a minimum to 12 hours in some cases.

If you have your last meal at night and don't eat anything until breakfast on the following day, you are effectively fasting. The good news here is that you are fasting, and you are not aware of it. If you split the word "breakfast" into two, it becomes "break" and "fast" which means that you are fasting and breaking the fast every single day.

Brilliant, isn't it? It is extremely empowering and liberating to know that you have been on the right track, well at least fifty percent on the right track all your life. As it is often said, that knowledge is power, in this case, the knowledge that you have been following a well-known eating practice is truly powerful.

All you need to know now is how to use the power that you already have and tweak it help you obtain optimal results.

Human beings have been following this eating pattern for ages now, and this is the only way that mankind knows. It is only in recent times that this age-old phenomenon has been repackaged as "intermittent fasting" and is being sold as a new technique, but in reality, this is the way we human beings have been living all our lives.

Now, you must be wondering why you are putting on weight or not reducing weight if you have been following this method all your life?

The answer is simple; it is because you were not doing it for a specific interval of time and consciously maintaining a schedule. Simply put in layman terms, it means fasting for a specific interval of time consistently to produce weight loss results.

So, what is the intermittent fasting about? It means that you fast for a period between 12-48 hours. The period when you are not eating is referred to as the fasting window. Whenever you break your fast, your eating window starts. Intermittent fasting fluctuates between the periods of eating and fasting. During the period of fast, you can consume liquids, if they don't contain any calories in them. When it comes to intermittent fasting, there are no hard and fast rules about what you can and cannot eat. In fact, this diet is completely customizable and has plenty of variations. You can tailor it to suit your needs based on your body type and health conditions. Those who practice this diet opt for a lifestyle that restricts their fasting window to 12-16 hours.

The biggest benefit of intermittent fasting is that you can choose a fasting window that fits your needs. You can make changes depending on how your body is responding to the fasting window. In all this, you are the owner of the process, and there are no stipulations or guidelines other than following a specific fasting window.

Truly, YOU are in charge of your makeover.

Chapter Two
History of Fasting

What makes intermittent fasting different than any other form of dieting is that it is not a modern fad; rather it is an age-old technique that has been rediscovered and brought back into the limelight by certain people. It is like Yoga of the world of food.

You will be surprised to know that people have been fasting since ancient days, perhaps right from the beginning of the human race. Really, if human bodies and evolution are to be taken into account, eating many meals and snacks throughout the day is neither necessary for survival, nor are they good for health. In fact excess of food, like the excess of anything can be extremely harmful to the body. In ancient times, the availability of food was unpredictable and irregular. It was difficult to gather and store food. Seasonal changes too made it difficult to come across food often. For instance, it was easy to get food in summers; however, it became excessively scarce in winters. This phenomenon of fluctuating food and food sources continued until the modern era for everyone except the upper class. In the last century, droughts, famines, wars, diseases, disorders, etc. led to the depletion of food sources. All of these led to starvation and sometimes death as well. It is no wonder that one of those famines is one of the Four Ushers of Apocalypse.

The history of fasting can be roughly divided into three eras - ancient, medieval and modern. Let us have a look at all three one by one.

Ancient History

The age of scrounging and gathering ended when humans discovered agriculture, perhaps by accident or observation. Once we discovered and developed agriculture, the incidents of famine went down. Agriculture led to the development of societies and culture and religion soon followed. Soon, people all over the world realized that going hungry for a limited period of time was actually beneficial for the health of your mind and body. This was then the first instance of periodic fasting. Periodic fasting became a staple of almost all the religions in the world. Forced starvation was replaced by controlled and voluntary fasting as it made people calm, happy and healthy. It is no wonder that fasting was often called 'detox' 'purification' 'purge' 'ritualistic cleaning' in ancient times. The ancients believed that fasting held the power to clean the body and the soul and that it could help them to please the God(s).

Spiritual Fasting

Religious or spiritual fasting still enjoys a strong position in all major religions. Buddha, Christ and Prophet Mohammad all believed in the power of fasting and advised their followers to fast periodically. It should be noted that fasting as a practice developed intrinsically and independently in varied cultures and religions. This means that people all over realized that fasting definitely had some benefits. Christians follow with Lent; Hindus with various different fasts and the Muslims followed Ramadan fasts. Similarly, the Buddhists and Jain came up with certain eating times that they must follow. All of these are types of fasting.

Fasting for Health in the Ancient Times

If we are to take into account the history of fasting for health benefits, we should be grateful to Ayurveda and the ancient Greeks. Ayurveda, I.e., the ancient medical science from India called for various forms of fasts and foods for different ailments and in general wellbeing. Hippocrates aka the father of Modern Medicine also wrote a lot about fasting and obesity. Obesity was on the rising in the times of Hippocrates in ancient Greek. This was due to the lavish lifestyle and lack of health routines for royalty. Hippocrates observed the correlation between obesity and early deaths and advised exercise and diet for obese people. The diet he advised included healthy food items and most prominently eating once a day only. After Hippocrates, Plutarch, the great historian too understood the importance of fasting. Great thinkers such as Plato and Aristotle followed this.

The ancient Greeks believed fasting could improve mental and cognitive abilities and thought it could help them solve problems and puzzles with ease. While this sounds a bit preposterous, try to imagine how bloated and uncomfortable you feel after having a large meal. Meals make you lethargic as your body focuses its energy on the digestive system. You feel excessively sleepy and often doze off after a heavy meal. Some people call this condition sleep coma. In contrast, if you avoid eating food for some time, you feel far more sharp, active and attuned to the atmosphere. Mind you this is no accident, it's an evolutionary effect. In the Stone Age, our senses became sharper when food was scarce.

Medieval Times

Even in the medieval times, the popularity of fasting did not wane, rather it continued to grow. Paracelsus, a Swiss-German physician who is well known as the father of toxicology, was a proponent of intermittent fasting. He was a firm believer of the theory that anything in excess can prove to be lethal and advised fasting for wellness. One of the founding fathers of the USA, Benjamin Franklin too was a proponent of intermittent fasting. A man of many talents, Franklin was a polymath who was well versed with many arts and sciences. Famous author Mark Twain too was a supporter of fasting for health.

Modern History of Fasting

While the rise of intermittent fasting, as a regular diet is a recent phenomenon, fasting, in general, continued its journey from medieval times to modern times. References to fasting can be found as early as the late 1800s. Interestingly fasting developed as a form of entertainment in the late 1800s and early 1900s. The fad died though- thankfully.

Fasting became a staple of medical literature around the early 1900s. Journal of Biological Chemistry defined fasting as a safe and effective way of losing weight and reducing obesity. However, obesity was perhaps the last thing on the minds of people in the early 20th century. The world was changing rapidly, and wars and famines had become commonplace. People were dying for epidemics and starvation all over. With the rise of obesity in the 21st century, fasting once again became popular.

Fasting and Evolution

Fasting was definitely a part of human evolution, and our body and mind are used and perhaps require regular periods of fasts. As most of the citizens of the developed and developing nations have access to ample food regularly, we have almost forgotten about fasting and it is no wonder that some people actually look down upon it. Still, intermittent fasting is becoming popular as more and more people see positive results.

Chapter Three
Why Intermittent Fasting

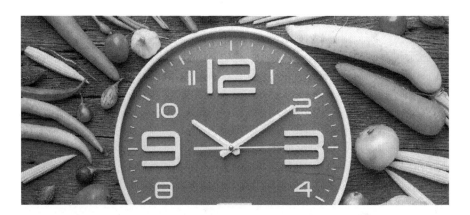

Contrary to popular belief, Intermittent Fasting is not a new age discovery or 21st-century invention made by scientists studying rats. It is a way of life that has been in existence since time immemorial.

Rather it is an ancient secret, almost like lost history that has only recently been excavated by scientists and so being tested on rats.

To begin with, early man or our predecessors before the age of internet or the age of even before the age of airplanes and cruise ships, human beings existed and therefore they had to eat because, despite all the modern advancements, the human body pretty much has remained the same, and therefore hunger has been constant. The early man had to go through long periods of fasting due to seasonal variations, drought or famine, and other natural calamities. Even when there were no natural calamities, food was never readily available, and every meal had to be sourced.

If you go back in time and rewind to tales of your parent's childhood or your grandparent's childhood, you will recollect how they never had access to leftover food. They always had fresh, simple meals made with ingredients found in their vicinity. This was the way of life until recently.

Have you wondered how before the advent of supermarkets or before the advent of refrigerators how did people eat? The answer to Intermittent Fasting lies in these questions because back in the day when there were no refrigerators and supermarkets, the humble human being lived the life of "hunter-gatherer." Living as a hunter-gatherer meant eating when one was able to gather food. When no food was available, they did not eat and yet the human species managed to survive.

The body has the wonderful capacity to store food in the form of fat and it uses these fat reserves when there is no additional fuel in the form of food being provided continuously without a break.

When the body starts using the fat reserves, there is no accumulation of weight, and therefore there was no concept of "Weight Loss." There was also no accumulation of weight because the early man had to first hunt for every meal because remember no refrigerator, which meant a lot of physical activity since there was no neighborhood supermarket where he or she could go to and procure food.

Technology and innovation changed the way humans have evolved. Industrialization completely changed the food industry. Factories started mushrooming during industrialization, and this introduced the concept of mass production of food. Mass production of food meant that markets are always flooded with food products. The concept of famine started to fade away slowly. After all, humans finally found a way to grow food with or without rainfall. All this changed the way human's view and consume food.

All the physical activity and the lack of access to food continuously meant that the human body would go into "fasting mode" from the "being fed" mode and use up the fat conserved.
Confusing right? But what do these terms "fasting mode" and "being fed mode," mean? It almost makes your body sound like a machine with various modes to function.

Being fed mode means continuously eating every few hours. This kind of lifestyle has been in vogue for the last few years where people have been encouraged to eat small meals every few hours. If you eat every few hours, your body is in the "fed" mode.

Fasting mode means when a person stops eating and has not fed the body anything for some time. These days the only time a person goes into fasting mode is while they are asleep.

So from a hunter-gatherer, man has come to a stage now where he or she is constantly in the fed mode. While the body is in the fed mode, it absorbs, digests and assimilates all the nutrients from the food being fed. In this state, it does not burn any energy or fat because it is constantly working to digest the food. It does not burn any fat because it depends on the nutrients present in the food being fed to provide the energy required for the functioning.

Since the body does not burn fat in the fed state, weight loss does not happen. Weight loss only happens when there is a caloric deficit, i.e. only when the body is not being fed and goes into fasting mode. Once the body enters fasting mode, it starts using the reserves of fat that it has stored away, and therefore weight loss happens. During the fasting state, the body burns fat reserves to provide energy for functioning.

Intermittent fasting is not a diet, but rather a way of life. It was the only way of life known to man before the industrial revolution took over society and supermarkets cropped up. Technological advancements have made it possible for fruit and vegetables to grow in all seasons, in all shapes and sizes. Technology has made it possible to store food for months together, and the mushrooming of online markets has made it possible to procure any food with one click and not leaving the confines of home.
But all this has also brought with it major health problems. While technological evolution has happened aggressively, biological evolution has not happened, and human beings have sadly not been able to catch up.

People often confuse "fasting" with "starvation" and use these words interchangeably. Contrary to popular belief, starvation and fasting are very different concepts. Fasting is a conscious decision to skip meals and not eat despite food being accessible. Starvation is involuntary when you want to eat but cannot because of food not being available and not knowing when the next meal will be available. By fasting and eventually feasting, it helps to consume food only during a specific time of the day and choose not to eat for a larger window of time.

The early man went through both periods of fasting and starvation. Consciously fasting has never killed a human being, whereas you have read about starvation leading to death. In the case of fasting food is accessible and the brain knows this. So there is no sense of fear and insecurity since you know that your next meal is available.

Centuries later, it is this concept that is being repackaged and sold as "Intermittent Fasting" to millions of people.

Intermittent fasting relies on the fundamental concept of moving the state of the body from the "being fed" mode to "fasting mode" and maintaining the fasting mode from anywhere between 8-16 hours.

You would "intermittently" eat during a short window of the day and "fast" during a larger window. Intermittent fasting is not a diet since you are eating!! It is not a starvation diet, but rather a healthy lifestyle. It is a way of living that you could sustain for the rest of your life.

Most importantly, intermittent fasting is one of the simplest strategies that we have for taking bad weight off with very little change to behavior and food choices. This is a good thing because human beings are by default creatures of habit and anything that requires a huge change to habits or behavior is not easily accepted.

The important word to remember is "fasting." This book will explain in detail:

- How intermittent fasting works
- The benefits of fasting
- The methods of fasting
- The demerits of fasting

To sum it up, intermittent fasting is simple enough that you will do, meaningful enough since it will make a difference.

How does Intermittent Fasting work?

The underlying principle for intermittent fasting is that it simply allows the body to burn off excess fat.

Your stomach secretes various enzymes that work rigorously on the food consumed, and post-digestion it turns into molecules in the bloodstream. Carbs in the form of refined grains (predominantly rice and white flour) become sugar, which is used by our cells for energy. Sugar can only enter our cells with the help of insulin, a hormone secreted by the pancreas. Insulin helps in transporting the sugar into the fat cells and keeps it there.

Insulin is the most important hormone that aids in the digestion and absorption of the food consumed and it is extremely sensitive to the different types of food. Insulin aids your body to use the sugar from the carbohydrates present in the food that has been consumed to be used as energy or to store it as fat for future use when the body is depleted of energy. Now comes the tricky part. The tricky part is that no matter what you eat, insulin levels will rise. All types of food will cause insulin levels to rise by a certain level. The key factor is to lower insulin levels or to ensure that insulin does not rise significantly.

How do we lower insulin levels when pretty much everything that is consumed increases the insulin? This is where the magical word "fasting" comes into focus. Fasting as it has always been called before making it intermittent fasting is an age-old tradition that has been followed by cultures across the world. It is one of the most ancient traditions in human history.

Between meals, if we skip snacks, our level of insulin will go become low which leads to the fat cells releasing stored sugar, as a means of energy. Weight loss is a result of lower levels of insulin. The idea behind intermittent fasting is to let the insulin levels go low and for a long time, so we burn off our fat, as insulin is the key hormone involved in the storage of food. Every time you eat, insulin rises to help to store the excess energy.

Now that you have been introduced to the terms feeding, fasting and insulin it is important to understand a fundamental question about how food gets digested and how does the body store the fat. Have you ever wondered how the body digests all the food we put into it? It is important to answer this question since it will help you understand the role fasting plays in digestion.

Your digestive system consists of a gastrointestinal tract called GI tract, liver, pancreas and gallbladder. For the purpose of simplifying the complex process of digestion, let us focus on the liver and pancreas. All the food that you consume is broken down into various components by the digestive system.

The protein breaks into amino acids, fats break into glycerol and fatty acids while carbohydrates break into sugar.

Insulin is a hormone secreted by the pancreas when you eat food. The pancreas releases insulin to help your body convert the sugars from the carbohydrates into glucose. Insulin is extremely sensitive to food and plays a vital role in turning the glucose into energy and distributing this energy to all the cells throughout the body. Post this distribution whatever is remained is then stored in the liver, muscle and fat cells to be used at a later stage when there is a shortage of energy. This excess that is stored is called glycogen. The body uses this glycogen during the fasting state or in between meals when there is no new food being consumed.

The pancreas also produces another secretion called glucagon. Insulin and glucagon work together to ensure the blood sugar balance is maintained. Both insulin and glucagon work in a negative feedback loop and trigger each other.

Glucagon comes into the picture in the fasting stage, as it counterbalances the work of insulin. After about six hours of consuming food, the glucose levels start decreasing in your bloodstream, and this triggers the pancreas to produce glucagon. The glucagon sends signals to the liver and the muscle cells to convert the stored glycogen into glucose and release it into the bloodstream so that other cells can use it for their energy needs.

This entire process is continuously happening in your body, therefore, ensuring the glucose levels are maintained and are under control.

It is this cycle that goes for a toss when you are in a constantly fed state. By being in a fed state for most of the time, you are not allowing your body to tap into the stored glycogen and help convert the glycogen to glucose. Once the natural rhythm of the body is disrupted, you start encountering health problems and from there on it's a road downhill. So, it is important to restore this natural rhythm to regain your health.

The exact reverse happens when you follow intermittent fasting. The reason for the reversal is that the insulin levels fall and send signals to the body to start burning stored energy. Once you stop feeding your body, it is forced to turn into the stored reserves as the body is naturally programmed to maintain the levels. Blood glucose falls, so the body has no choice but to pull glucose out of storage to burn for energy. It turns to glycogen since it is readily available and works on converting it to energy. It is broken down to provide energy for the other cells. The energy therefore obtained can fuel the body for anywhere between 24 hours to 36 hours. Post this; the body will break down the stored fat for energy.

All this teaches an important and simple lesson and that is that the body exists in two states, i.e. fed and fasted. As long as the fed and the fasting states are in balance, there will be no issues.

If we start eating the minute we get out of bed, and do not stop until we go to sleep, we spend almost all our time in the fed state. Over time, we will gain weight. We have not allowed our body at any time to burn food energy. Which means there is no downtime where the body can focus on utilizing the stored fats. Over a period of time, this fat accumulation becomes too much and starts showing up externally on the stomach, thighs, arms and just about anywhere and internally the fat gets stored around the organs such as the liver and clogs the arteries.

The external appearance of fat might make you feel ugly and undesirable, but the real problem lies with the internal fat also called visceral fat. It is this excess fat that clogs the arteries that lead to heart problems and other severe life threating diseases.

Simply put, intermittent fasting allows your body to work because you are providing it rest by not continuously feeding it. When you constantly feed the body, it must first work on processing the new food vs. trying to work on the reserves. By constantly working the reserves keep increasing and are never used. Since this extra energy is not tapped, it shows up on the weighing scale and on various parts of our body. Hopefully, by now you know how you developed love handles and not biceps or the secret behind your sagging tummy.

The following sections and chapters will help you understand how to tackle your tummy and become fit from fat.

Why is it easy to burn fat while fasting?

The secret is that insulin levels are low when fasting. When you are in a fasted state, your body can burn fat that has been inaccessible during the fed state.

The reason the body cannot access the stored reserves is that we do not enter the fasting state until about 6- 12 hours after the last meal, it's rare that our bodies are in the fat burning state. Fasting forces your body to go into a fat burning mode, something that you rarely get into when on feeding mode.

Fasting state leaves no stone unturned in ensuring that the excess fat is used because the body does not have access to a recently consumed meal to work or to tap energy from, so it is more likely to turn to the fat reserves stored in your body as it is the only energy reserve readily available. On a normal eating schedule, insulin levels are always at a high, and therefore any additional food you put into the body will be stored as fat.

Intermittent fasting is all about educating your body about the reserves of energy available, guiding it to use the consumed food more efficiently, and helping your body to use fat as fuel when we deprive it of new food to constantly work on.

It is fascinating to know that the human body has well-developed mechanisms to deal with periods of low availability of food and is extremely adaptable. To put it in simple words, intermittent fasting is the process of switching the body from burning glucose (which is readily available) to burning fat (which is not readily available). When the body is depleted of food, stored food is naturally released.

Intermittent fasting is one of the most efficient ways to ensure that low insulin levels are maintained, as blood glucose levels remain normal when the body switches to burning fat that has been stored.

Lowering the insulin levels will also cause the body to get rid of excess water and salt, and the body stops retaining water.

What makes Intermittent Fasting different?

In today's day and age, you really have to be living under a rock if you cannot name at least 2 diets that some neighbor or co-worker has been following.

Add to the confusion of the already existing diets that make no sense, every day a new diet pops up. There is always some new diet that social media influencers are talking about and crediting to their marvelous transformation. This "discovery" or "invention" of a new diet is often accompanied by a stream of recipes that call for unheard of ingredients that not only will burn a hole in your pocket but also are quite difficult to follow for someone who is still reeling from the after-effects of the previous diet.

If you are someone who can relate to the above experience, then you are not alone in this battle. Intermittent fasting is for people like you, who have religiously followed every diet under the sun, can identify the different types of sugars, and can instantly spot the difference between authentic organic food and inorganic food but yet have not lost a single pound of weight.

Here in lies the beauty of intermittent fasting. It does not require you to be a chef, neither does it burn a hole in your pocket and leave your pantry with a plethora of ingredients that have never been used before. Intermittent fasting is a simple process for simple people like you and me who want to change their lives and become better genuinely.
It is uncomplicated, easy and can be followed with slight modifications to your existing lifestyle because you are already

aware that you fast. What is special or different about intermittent fasting as compared to the plethora of diets floating around?

Lifestyle modification:

To begin with, intermittent fasting advocates lifestyle modification. A random Google search about intermittent fasting will tell you that it is not a diet, to begin with, as it comes with no recommendations about the type of foods to eliminate or the type of foods to focus on. Intermittent fasting does not have any guidelines about food groups and does not ask the follower to give up on any food group. Most, if not all the other diets are difficult to follow because they start with asking people to give up on certain food groups completely. This becomes very difficult for the average person to follow and so people completely stop following it. It is important to remember that giving up on an entire food group is not possible and neither is it sustainable in the long run.

Customizable:

It empowers the follower, i.e. you by letting you decide what works for you and does not work for you. Other diets place a lot of restrictions on followers by having strict do's and don'ts. They place a huge emphasis on counting macros, using certain ingredients while forbidding others while cooking, etc. At times certain ingredients that other diets call for might not be available in your place of residence or might be expensive. Intermittent fasting does not come with any such pre-requisites. It does not recommend specific cooking methodology, special ingredients and neither does it forbid anything. The only emphasis is on "fasting", and it lets you decide when to fast and for "how long" you can fast.

Does not guarantee immediate results:

I know that this can be quite disheartening to read, but it is important to understand that nothing happens overnight and that consistency is the key if you want to see results that last and not vanish just as quickly as they came. Unlike other diets on the market, intermittent fasting DOES NOT guarantee results within a finite timeline. This is a very important thing to know and understand because it is a lifestyle modification and such modifications take time. Intermittent fasting is a habit that needs to be inculcated and nurtured in order to see results.

For e.g., if you are looking for a quick fix solution to fit into a dress two sizes less than your current size within a week, then this not for you.

Intermittent fasting is akin to growing a tree. Just like it takes time, care and nurturing for a seed to grow into a tree, intermittent fasting takes commitment to show results. It is about developing a relationship with yourself, planning and sticking to it.

Triggers hormonal adaptations:

Fasting triggers numerous hormonal modifications that DO NOT happen with other diets. Insulin drops precipitously, and the metabolism rate rises. When the body is in fasting mode, it opens up to the reserves of fat stored and uses it. Basal metabolism stays high and changes fuel sources from food, to stored food or body fat. During fasting, glycogen is burned first, and when that is finished, the body turns to the fat stored. Other diets do not focus on balancing insulin. Apart from insulin, intermittent fasting also helps in regulating other hormonal fluctuations, which will be discussed in detail in the further chapters of this book.

Focuses on reducing visceral fat:

Visceral fat is the most dangerous fat as it surrounds organs such as the liver. It is the visceral fat that is more dangerous as compared to the fat that is seen externally, and the reason for this has been discussed above. Intermittent fasting has shown to reduce this type of fat effectively as compared to other diets that focus on calorie restriction.

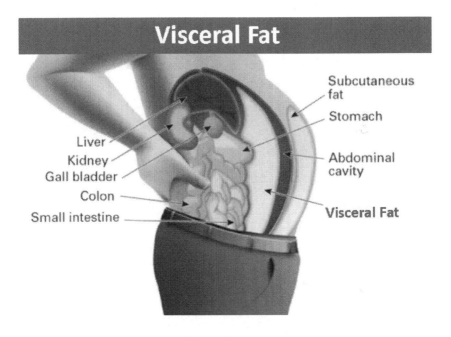

Chapter Four
Other Diets Often Fail

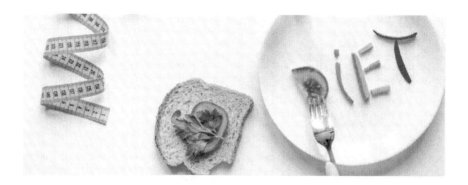

One of the major problems with other diets is that they are extremely difficult to follow. While most of them do work, it becomes very difficult to follow them especially if you have a hectic schedule.

Two major reasons why people diet is type 2 diabetes and obesity. Diets are highly effective in both these conditions. Low carb diet is best for people who have Type 2 diabetes. A diet that is high in protein can also prove to be beneficial for such people as protein stimulates the production of insulin. So, patients of type 2 diabetes should ideally follow a diet that is low in carbohydrates, high in protein and that does not contain a lot of processed foods, including sugar. While this sounds easy on paper, it is quite difficult to follow such a diet and adhere to it religiously in today's world. People tend to find loopholes in the diet, as controlling your taste buds is a difficult task. For instance, if a diet asks a person to avoid dairy, they may start consuming non-dairy milk such as almond milk, soymilk, etc. While these kinds of milk have comparatively fewer calories, it will still mess up the diet plan. We become habitual of our daily diet, which makes it difficult to adopt any new one.

Continuing the case of Type 2 diabetes patients, it has been proven that a low-carb diet can really keep the disorder under control. This is where intermittent fasting comes on the scene. In intermittent fasting, your meal remains the same only the time of meals becomes restricted. Fasting can help people to cut carbs from their meals with ease.

Intermittent fasting is an excessively simple way of following a healthy diet routine. When people are advised to eat healthily, they often get confused, as even in the era of smartphones it is difficult to follow a diet plan to the T and check the nutritional value of all the food that you consume throughout the day. As there exists a variety of diets such as low carb, low fat, low sugar, low calorie, etc. It becomes very difficult to follow any one of them without causing some sort of confusion. In contrast, intermittent fasting is not only simple to perform but easy to remember as well. In fact, it can be summed up in a sentence. 'While fasting, avoid eating anything except water, bone broth or black tea/coffee.' That's all you need to remember while following an intermittent fasting diet.

Certain fad diets fail because they are not healthy or do not have any scientific backing. Other diets fail because people cannot follow them. Intermittent fasting works because it is backed by science and is easy to follow.

It is Free

Being healthy is not cheap, especially in today's world where everything has become a commodity, and every field has become an industry. Health is an industry where fit and healthy looking individuals are the commodities. To achieve a healthy body, it is necessary to eat organic and live a healthy lifestyle. But eating organic is not cheap and is not a viable option for many. Not everyone can afford local, unprocessed bread and grass-fed beef. It has been observed that healthy and organic foods cost ten times as much as junk or processed foods. While eating on a budget, you will definitely think about money before thinking of whether an item is organic or not.

Many diets recommend organic and natural foods. Not all people can afford to follow these diets. This is why fasting is one of the best diets because not only is it free, but it may save your hard earned money as well! When you cut-off certain meals from your diet, you will save some cash at the end of the month.

You do not need to spend money on supplements, healthy and organic foods, shakes, protein bars, etc. While fasting, therefore making it the most convenient form of dieting.

Convenience

Another highly recommended dietary habit is cooking your own, fresh meal every time you want to eat something. Not many people like to cook and consider it to be a time wasting task. After all, why cook when you can buy much tastier food in no time from a restaurant? Not everyone has the time to cook every day. Everyone is on a tight schedule nowadays and incorporating all the pre and post cooking activities in such a schedule is almost impossible. Cooking involves a lot of pre-planning such as shopping, looking for a recipe, preparation for the recipe, etc. Then once you are done with cooking, you need to clean away the mess caused while cooking. This is why the number and frequency of people eating out have been increasing steadily since the last few years.

Forcing people to cook at home does not work, and people will always try to find loopholes. Fasting can help such people who want to eat healthily and follow a diet while being on a tight budget and schedule. Fasting needs no preparation like shopping, and you don't have to clean up anything afterward. It's as easy as it gets.

No Cravings

What comes to your mind when you think of dieting? Most of the people think of cutting-off snacks, parties, desserts, etc. Many diets do advise people to avoid ice creams, snacks, desserts, etc. Forever. While this is thoroughly sound advice, it is impractical and difficult to follow. You can cut-off desserts for a couple of months, and for some people a year or two, but imagine cutting-off dessert for the rest of your life. Sounds preposterous, right? Imagine going to a wedding or a birthday and not enjoying the cake. Or going to a party and avoiding alcohol. Or going to Thanksgiving dinner and avoiding everything but the salad. You will become healthy - but your life will become dull. Fasting can help you with this.

Of course, fasting does not mean that you can eat desserts and snacks for every meal every day. You still need to keep an eye on proportions and eat a balanced diet. You can have desserts and snacks on certain days while fasting. You can feast, but you must fast later. Fasting is a flexible form of diet, and you can manipulate it according to your needs. For instance, if you need to visit a party, you can break your fast; however, you must fast after the party. It is all about balance, fasting and feasting should go hand in hand.

Fasting is a lifestyle

Fasting is not a fad diet, and rather it is a change that you incorporate in your day-to-day life. You can fast until you see your desired results or can fast until you want. It will keep you energized and feel healthy. It is definitely one of the most powerful methods of weight loss. It is also extremely flexible and it can be combined with other diets. Certain diets such as the Paleo diet, ketogenic diet, low-carb diet, etc. are very compatible with fasting.

You make your own diet plans while fasting. For instance, certain diets call for eating as soon as you wake up and then continue eating after every two hours. This sort of diet is extremely intrusive and disruptive. Fasting, however, can be done anytime you want. It has no set period or duration. It has no fixed pattern, and you can adjust it according to your needs. For instance, you may fast twice a week for your first week and may increase or decrease the days for the second.

If you fall sick or do not feel well, you can stop fasting. The results won't go away. You can even stop for several weeks for medical or any other reasons.

Compatibility

As said earlier, fasting is extremely compatible with other diets. There are certain diets that allow users to consume only specific food items. For instance, the Paleo diet calls for meat-based products while a low carb diet asks you to avoid processed foods. Fasting has no such restrictions. If you are a regular meat eater, you can still fast. If you are allergic to gluten, you can still fast. As you are only changing when you eat and not what you eat, it does not matter whether you don't want to eat something. Fasting will allow you to do so. Therefore fasting has multiple advantages over regular diets.

Chapter Five
Does Intermittent Fasting Work the Same Way for Men and Women?

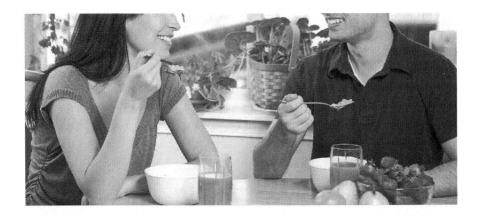

As far as intermittent fasting and women are concerned, it a love-hate kind of relationship. There is some evidence that states that intermittent fasting does help women especially those diagnosed with problems such as Polycystic Ovarian Syndrome (PCOS) and insulin resistance.

There are many narratives from women who complained of a change in their menstrual cycles after practicing intermittent fasting. These changes happen because a woman's body is extremely sensitive towards calorie restriction.

The effects of fasting ultimately come down to human biology. Since men and women are biologically different, the impact of fasting also differs. It has been observed that while shorter periods of fasting are generally safe, extended periods of fasting have shown to cause disruptions to women's hormones causing issues such as reproductive problems and early onset of menopause.

Hormones are vital for the functioning of the human body and play a very important role in ovulation. The reproductive functions such as ovulation are controlled and regulated by an area in the brain called as hypothalamus which contains sensors that can determine the levels of energy the body has access to from the food being consumed. Depending on the levels of energy, the sensors initiate signals on whether to create or conserve energy.

Research has shown that there are certain special types of neurons in the hypothalamus called kisspeptin that control the release of a hormone called gonadotrophin. The primary function of the gonadotropins is to indicate to the pituitary gland to produce two hormones called the Luteinizing hormone (LH) and the follicular stimulating hormone (FSH) hormones which in turn signal the ovaries to produce estrogen and progesterone.

It has been found in rats, that this wonderful system goes for a toss during acute metabolic stress. This research has been extended to a female body to suggest that during situations of metabolic stress, the body does not adapt properly and so ovulation gets disrupted.

Apart from hormonal fluctuations, the other reason fertility issues occur is that when the female body senses the fasting state; it assumes there is starvation. The body cannot differentiate between "fasting" which is a voluntary action and "starvation" which is an involuntary action.

When the female body senses the alternation to the normal eating schedule, the hormone levels ghrelin and leptin are affected. These are the hunger hormones, which when affected increase hunger pangs signaling to eat. This can easily trigger a woman to binge eat to compensate for the hunger and then restrict food completely. This irregular pattern disrupts the hormones.

Fasting interferes with ovulation since the female body senses the unavailability of food causing the hormones to shift in a manner that disrupts ovulation. Biologically, when the body senses starvation it simply understands that the time is not right to get pregnant. This is the body's natural way of protecting a potential pregnancy even if you are not trying to conceive.

Hormones are extremely sensitive to even the slightest changes, and all of them are interconnected. So, when one of them gets disrupted, the effect trickles down, and the rest follow suit. This is like the "domino effect."

In order to not disrupt the natural rhythm of the hormones, women need to tread with caution when trying intermittent fasting. While prolonged periods of fasting have not yielded positive results, it is a widely known fact that PCOS, insulin resistance causes weight gain, which can lead to infertility. All this shows that a proper balance needs to be maintained. Intermittent fasting for short periods of time might indeed be the solution to the problem. Prolonged periods of fasting and aggressive methods might not yield positive results. They might disrupt the entire system and cause unintended damage to the body.

Women should, therefore, adopt a revised approach toward intermittent fasting. They should consider fewer fasting days and shorter fasting periods. When done within a brief timeframe, intermittent fasting can help you reach your weight loss goals without disrupting your hormones.

But why does intermittent fasting affect some women in a negative manner?

There is very little research that is available to deduce specific results on this matter as scientists have only recently begun to study intermittent fasting and its effects. There is no concrete answer available yet to understand the negative implications of intermittent fasting. The negative factors have been attributed to kisspeptin by some studies as it has already been established about the role kisspeptin plays in facilitating the production of estrogen. It has also been found that kisspeptin is extremely dependent on other hormones and therefore any changes in hormones that impact hunger can cause the kisspeptin levels to rise. So it has been advised that women do not fast for prolonged periods of time since it's a very delicate balance that goes out of sync.

It has been identified that the quantity of protein consumed by women is lesser than when compared to men. Therefore, it is quite natural that the protein consumption of a woman will further reduce during fasting. In the previous section related to digestion, it has been established that proteins are converted to amino acids during the process of digestion. Amino acids are essential to stimulate estrogen, and for the synthesis of IGF1 (a growth factor-like insulin), that is released by the liver. This hormone released by the liver is responsible for the thickening of the uterine lining and helps with the reproductive cycle. Therefore, any diet that is low in protein can adversely affect fertility. It helps to understand that estrogen is an important hormone not just for reproduction but for various other functions too. Women have estrogen receptors present throughout their bodies, and they are even present in the brain. Therefore, any change in the estrogen levels can cause a change in the metabolism of the body. Apart from ovulation and reproductive functions, estrogen is also known to influence the cognitive functions, moods and bone health in women. Estrogen also regulates your appetite and energy levels. Estrogen alters peptides in the brainstem that indicate whether you are hungry or not.

Estrogen also stimulates the neurons present in the hypothalamus that control the production of peptides. A decline in estrogen levels increases hunger pangs and promotes binge eating. So, it is safe to assume that estrogens are essential for metabolic regulation in the body. The ratio of various estrogenic metabolites like estradiol, estrone, and estriol varies over time. Before the onset of menopause, the primary type of estrogen is estradiol. Once you hit menopause, the levels of estradiol decrease while the level of estrone stays the same, it is not yet clear as to the role that these different estrogens play in the body. A general theory is that a decrease in estradiol can increase fat retention in the body. This happens because estradiol is important to synthesize fats and any decrease in this level reduces your body's ability to process fats. Therefore, it is quite common that women who have hit menopause often struggle with losing weight.

All this might sound scary and intimidate you. If you are a woman reading this, you might even wonder if you will ever reach your weight goals. When you encounter such thoughts, it is important to remember that most of the research that is available today on intermittent fasting has been conducted on rats. There is little research that has been done on human beings, and the verdict on this is not yet fully out there.

In fact, some recent studies claim that there are benefits to intermittent fasting in a certain section of women who are suffering from hormonal disorders such as PCOS or insulin resistance.

Benefits for women:

On the other hand, some recent research has also suggested that intermittent fasting might prove to be beneficial for women who are suffering from PCOS.

Most women suffering from PCOS have insulin resistance and the reverse also can be possible where insulin resistance in some women might cause PCOS. PCOS, in turn, causes infertility in women.

Since intermittent fasting has shown to be good at managing insulin levels, it might also be helpful in managing PCOS as a result of good insulin control.
A recent study published in 2017 states that since fasting has shown to manage glucose and insulin levels and reduce weight, it could consequently have a beneficial effect on ovarian function and infertility in PCOS women.

Reduce inflammation: Intermittent fasting has also shown a reduction in inflammation that can help reduce weight and resolve PCOS issues to a large extent.

The road ahead for women

Given all the information that has been presented so far, it is natural to wonder about what lies ahead for you if you are a female reading this.
With all the drawbacks mentioned, you may be wondering if this is the right way to proceed and whether you could still follow it and not disrupt your body.

Based on all the information available so far, it is safe to say that you must be very cautious while following the protocols of intermittent fasting. As with everything in life, moderation is the key. Whenever you opt for this diet, you must opt for a balanced, relaxed approach and test waters for the first few days so that it will not stress your body. There are various changes that take place in your body when you follow the protocols of intermittent fasting. A healthy adult can safely adhere to the principles of intermittent fasting.

There are a couple of things that you must keep in mind while following intermittent fasting.

If you experience any of the following symptoms, you must stop the diet immediately and consult a medical practitioner.

The symptoms that you need to watch out for are any irregularities in menstruation, lack of sleep, hair fall, dry skin or acne. Other symptoms include extreme tiredness and a decline in your recovery time. If you notice extreme mood swings or a decline in your sex drive, then it is time to stop intermittent fasting and consult a medical practitioner.

As with all dietary modifications and interventions, it is important to consult your doctor anytime you have a suspicion. Prevention is always better than cure and more so in the case where health is involved.

Chapter Six:
Who should Avoid Fasting?

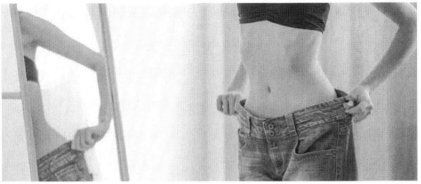

Intermittent fasting definitely has a lot of benefits and is definitely one of the best diets you can follow, but there is a caveat- fasting is not meant for everyone. Yes, not everyone can and should fast, as it may prove disastrous. There are certain conditions in which fasting is not recommended.

Certain people should absolutely avoid fasting. These include:

Underweight or malnourished people

Underweight undernourished people or those on the verge of malnutrition should not fast. If you are concerned about malnutrition or believe that you are underweight, then you need to steer clear from fasting.

As said above, when your body fat levels are under 4% your body starts using muscles and proteins as a source of energy. Your body starts burning functional tissues to survive, and it starts to 'waste' itself. This is an extremely dangerous condition that may lead to lifelong problems or even death.

To check whether fasting is suitable for you or not, just check your BMI. While not a foolproof science, BMI or Body Mass Index is a good way of checking whether you are overweight/underweight.

BMI is calculated by dividing your weight in kilograms by your height in meter squared. If your BMI is under 18.5, then you are underweight, and you should avoid fasting. People whose BMI is around 20 should ideally avoid fasting as well unless recommended by a certified health professional.

Anorexia

People who suffer from anorexia should definitely avoid fasting. Anorexic people are often already malnourished, and fasting will just put additional stress on their bodies. Food is like medicine for anorexics and withholding it may lead to disastrous results.

It should be noted that fasting does not lead to anorexia. Anorexia is a psychiatric disorder, and under eating has no hand in its development.

Fasting is not addictive. Saying that fasting causes anorexia is like saying that washing your hands causes OCD. Undereating is a symptom of anorexia and not a cause.

Fasting has a history of thousands of years while anorexia is a new phenomenon. As it is impossible to find any depiction of anorexia in ancient times, it is safe to assume that fasting does not cause it.

Children

Children need a lot of nutrition for the overall proper development of their mind and body. This nutrition is achieved from food. Therefore, restricting food can have long-term negative effects on children. Adequate nutrition is absolutely necessary for normal growth in children. If children do not receive ample nutrition, the development of their vital organs including the brain, etc. may not happen properly. Underfeeding in the teenage years can also cause a variety of problems. Teenage years are the years when puberty takes place, and puberty like any other developmental and growth spurt requires a lot of energy and nutrients.

While missing a few meals will not hinder the development, children are advised against fasting for longer durations. Instead of fasting, children should try to learn the importance of nutrition and healthy eating. If your children love eating junk food, try to help them to switch over to healthier alternatives.

Pregnancy

This should come as a no-brainer. A woman's body needs a lot of nutrients to ensure proper development of the fetus. Without adequate nutrients, the fetus may develop abnormalities that can prove to be life-threatening for the mother and the baby. Pregnant women require specially enriched diets and often a dietary supplement to ensure their and their baby's health. Therefore, cutting down on food can prove to be disastrous.

People who are on medication

People who take regular medications should avoid fasting altogether or should contact a physician before starting a fast. Certain medications cannot and should not be taken on an empty stomach as they may lead to various side effects. Common medicines that may cause side effects while fasting includes aspirin, iron supplements, magnesium supplements, metformin, etc.

Diabetes

Yes, while fasting can be quite beneficial to people who have diabetes; you should not start fasting without contacting a doctor first. Diabetes, whether type 1 or 2, is a high-risk disorder that should not be taken for granted. Never change your diet without contacting a health professional first. Your medicines may cause problems with your blood sugar levels if you start a diet suddenly. Your blood sugar level may go down drastically. This condition is known as hypoglycemia. Symptoms of hypoglycemia include sweating, shaking, nervousness, irritability, hunger, nausea, feeling faint, etc. In severe cases, hypoglycemia may lead to delirium, confusion, seizures, etc. In extreme cases, it may cause death. If you ever feel these symptoms, ingest some sugary products as soon as possible.

GERD

GERD of gastroesophageal reflux disease is a common disease that leads to stomachache, heartburn, acid reflux, etc. It often causes pain in the chest and nausea. Fasting can make this problem severe. It is recommended to contact a physician before starting a fast.

Women

Women can fast; however, there are certain things that you need to keep in mind before fasting. You will find more information regarding this later in the book.

If you have an already identified medical condition or suspect any changes to your health, you should consult your doctor before starting intermittent fast.

This is especially true if you:

- Have diabetes
- Have problems with blood sugar regulation
- Low blood pressure
- Are currently on medications
- Underweight
- History of eating disorders
- Are a woman trying to conceive
- Are pregnant or breastfeeding
- Have a history of amenorrhea

Well, if you have lasted so long despite all the heavy-duty learning about insulin, glycogen, and glucagon, then I can safely assume that you have indeed committed to transforming yourself.

Congratulations on taking that first big step. Armed with all this knowledge, you now enter into the next phase, which is the implementation phase. All this knowledge that you have acquired will be of no use if you do not know the benefits of the knowledge.

Knowledge is available relatively easily these days and pretty much every person has some amount of it. Sadly, knowing does not produce results on its own. Read on to know what to do with all the newly acquired knowledge and transform yourself.

Chapter Seven
Benefits of Intermittent Fasting

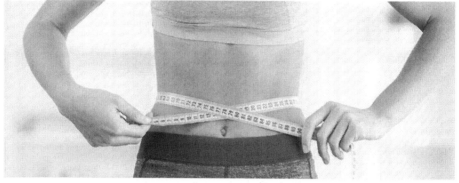

Before you embark on this wonderful journey of becoming "Flab to Fab" and "Fat to Fit," it is important that you know the benefits of intermittent fasting. So here they are.

Weight Loss

The one thing that almost all the scientists who have spent a better part of their lives researching intermittent fasting agree is that almost all forms of intermittent fasting have shown to reduce weight. This has been mentioned in a study conducted in 2015 that almost 13 intervention trials that were studied concluded that intermittent fasting does cause weight loss.

In the same study, it has also been mentioned that the amount of weight loss though depends on what kind of intermittent fasting intervention or method was followed.

Brain functioning

According to a study conducted by neuroscientist Mark Mattson, fasting not only impacted the waistline but it also had a positive impact on the functioning of the brain.

In the above article, Mattson mentions that in studies conducted by his team they found that intermittent fasting by limiting calorie intake for at least two days in a week helped neural connections in the hippocampus while protecting neurons against accumulation of amyloid plaques, a form of protein that is predominantly present in patients suffering from Alzheimer's disease.

In a study on mice, intermittent fasting showed improved performance on measures of cognitive decline that are associated with aging.

Another study done on intermittent fasting has shown to protect memory and learning functionality as well.

Longevity

Intermittent fasting research on animals has shown a direct correlation between the restriction of calories that lead to fewer diseases and thereby increasing lifespan.

Insulin Growth factor is a hormone that is linked to certain diseases such as cancer and diabetes that have shown to decrease lifespan. Few experts on this topic are of the opinion that eating increases the insulin growth factor since any food consumed increases insulin levels. So fasting is the way to reduce insulin levels that could lower the risk for contracting these life threating diseases and increase lifespan.

Cancer

As you have read above, that the food consumed has a direct impact on the production of insulin growth factor, the hormone that seems to be responsible for causing diseases such as cancer. So, fasting which will reduce insulin automatically lowers the risk for cancer by impacting the growth of certain kinds of tumors.

Another study conducted on a small size among people has shown that intermittent fasting significantly reduced the side effects of chemotherapy (a very popular form of cancer treatment) such as nausea, fatigue, and diarrhea.

Disclaimer: It is important to remember that intermittent fasting should not be done if you are already a cancer patient without the guidance of your physician. If you are a cancer patient or know anyone who is a cancer patient and is keen on trying intermittent fasting, it is not advisable to do it unless supervised by a physician.

Blood sugar

Intermittent fasting has a huge benefit since it directly tackles the problem with elevated insulin levels. In the preceding chapters, you have learned how insulin is the main hormone that makes or breaks everything in your body at least as far as food is concerned. While all hormones control bodily functions, insulin is very powerful since it has a direct impact on other hormones such as estrogen, progesterone and also on the brain. It has been proven consistently that intermittent fasting whether short term or long term significantly lower insulin levels therefore automatically regulating other hormones and improving the blood sugar level. Elevated blood sugar is life threating, and this can be controlled by following intermittent fasting.

Physiological benefits

Several theories provide the reason as to why fasting provides physiological benefits. One of the theories is that fasting causes mild stress to the cells. You are depleting the cells of ready energy by not providing food continuously. Depletion of energy causes mild stress in the cells, and the cells respond to this stress by adapting to it. The body is naturally made to cope with stress and resist diseases.

Contrary to popular belief, some amount of stress is good for the body. If you think about it, stressing the body is using the body such as when you exercise you stress the muscles and the cardiovascular system. When you work on your laptop, you are using your mind and therefore causing stress to it. But this kind of stress is good since it helps your body grow fitter and stronger. It is this lack of stress completely that is causing a lot of problems today.

As long as you give your body the time to recover and learn, it will grow and serve you. Intermittent fasting has also shown to have the same kind of effect on cells that exercise has.

Type 2 Diabetes

Intermittent fasting curbs insulin resistance thereby lowering your risk for getting Type 2 Diabetes, as it is caused by elevated blood sugar levels. Intermittent fasting reduces insulin levels, which help to control blood sugar thereby reducing your risk of getting Type 2 diabetes.

In studies done on humans, intermittent fasting has shown to reduce blood sugar levels significantly.

It is extremely important to control blood sugar levels because an increase in blood sugar not only causes type 2 diabetes but also a plethora of other diseases. Type 2 diabetes is a disease that has no cure so far and can only be managed. It is just the tip of the iceberg because if not managed well, type2 diabetes can lead to diseases such as kidney failure, eye problems, and cardiovascular diseases as well.

A study conducted on diabetic rats has shown that intermittent fasting protected against kidney damage, which is one of the most common and severe complications associated with diabetes.

Disclaimer: If you already have diabetes, then you should not start intermittent fasting without consulting your physician. All the information mentioned above is written for people to lower their risk of getting diabetes but not intended for someone already diagnosed with it.

An entire section has also been devoted to the effects of intermittent fasting on women. If you are a woman with diabetes, it is all the more important that you consult a physician before attempting to begin intermittent fasting.

Inflammation and Oxidative Stress

Oxidative stress involves molecules called free radicals that are highly unstable that react with other molecules and cause damage to the body.

A lot of studies have revealed that intermittent fasting reduces oxidative stress considerably thereby reducing the damage caused by free radicals by enhancing the body's resistance to oxidative stress.

Inflammation is another key problem that is the cause of several diseases such as PCOS. Intermittent fasting is known to tackle this problem by reducing inflammation and thereby lowering the risk of getting diseases such as PCOS.

Heart Health

Intermittent fasting can be extremely beneficial for the health of your heart. The health of your heart is associated with various health markers or risk factors such as blood pressure, blood sugar levels, cholesterol levels, i.e. HDL and LDL, blood triglycerides. Obesity is the most common cause of heart problems since it leads to the buildup of plaque and clogs the arteries. Stress, inflammation or diabetes worsens this condition. Intermittent fasting helps combat this problem since it helps in insulin regulation and weight loss by burning fat and therefore reducing the formation of plaque. This also helps to maintain other health markers such as cholesterol, blood pressure within their limit and therefore improve heart health leading to an overall improvement in health.

Cellular repair process: Intermittent fasting is supposed to promote a process called "Autophagy."

Autophagy is defined as the process of the natural, regulated mechanism of the cell that disassembles itself of the unnecessary or dysfunctional components. This process was related to starvation but off late a lot of research is being done to see whether intermittent fasting also promotes autophagy.

It is fascinating that the human body already has a mechanism where it conveniently disposes of the unnecessary components similar to waste removal. Autophagy allows this degeneration to be done in an orderly manner and allows for the recycling of the components as well. It has been found that in cases of extreme starvation, this process of autophagy kicks in and is responsible for the breakdown of cellular components to promote cellular survival by ensuring that energy levels are maintained.

Recent studies have revealed that intermittent fasting also promotes cellular regeneration, therefore, reducing the likelihood of contracting diseases and increasing lifespan.

In 2016, a Japanese scientist Yoshinori Ohsumi won the Nobel Prize for his research related to autophagy. Since then diet and wellness experts are claiming that intermittent fasting also induces autophagy. Increased autophagy is considered to protect against diseases such as Alzheimer's and cancer.

Sleep

If you are overweight or have put on a lot of weight recently you might observe that your sleep patterns have changed, as obesity and excess weight are known to cause sleep problems. When your body does not get enough rest that it needs, then your internal fat burning mechanism takes a backseat. Intermittent fasting helps regulate your sleep cycle by working on improving the efficiency of burning fat. A good sleep cycle has physical and psychological effects. You will feel energetic and refreshed if you get enough sleep.

Gut health

Intermittent fasting promotes good gut health. Are you aware that your body is home to many microbes? Yes, that's right. Your body is home to many microbes, and these are not to be confused with the microbes that are bad and cause infections. Rather, these microbes present in your gut specifically aid in digesting the food that is consumed. They are good bacteria that are needed for the optimal functioning of your gut. Your gut is home to millions of microorganisms.

The food that you consume has a direct impact on these bacteria. Food consumed can change the microbe communities although the research about how it changes is still not conclusive. You might be surprised to know that not just "what" you eat impacts the gut health but also "when" you eat has an impact. This is where intermittent fasting comes into the picture because it is all about specific periods of fasting that intermittent fasting focuses on.
Scientific research done mostly on animals has shown to improve the microbe diversity of the gut with intermittent fasting and increase the tolerance to the bad bacteria.

Intermittent fasting helps improve the health of these microbes. When these microbes are functioning well, then it improves your body's ability to digest as well as absorb food. Intermittent fasting has also shown to protect the gut against the negative impact of stress that includes inflammation.

Some amount of early research also states that periods of fasting allow the gut to rest and therefore helps in restoring the intestinal walls. This is of paramount importance as it protects against a "leaky gut" or gut permeability, which is a process that is facilitated by diets that are high in fats. The high-fat diets allow bad bacteria and other toxins to enter the surrounding tissues in the gut, which causes inflammation.

Therefore, intermittent fasting can theoretically increase low insulin levels by promoting insulin sensitivity, enhance immune tolerance, reduce inflammation and promote the renewal of cells. All these ultimately promote good health that leads to a longer life.

Blood pressure

Research has shown that intermittent fasting helps maintain blood pressure effectively. It has been found that participants who followed intermittent fasting cleared fat from their body quickly and also reported a nine percent drop in the systolic pressure.

Energetic and Focused

Have you ever noticed how after eating a heavy meal full of carbohydrates, you do not feel energetic at all? How many times have you struggled to focus on doing simple tasks that otherwise require no energy but after a heavy meal seem like a burden? How many times were you caught sleeping or yawning during meetings after lunch? This happens because the food, contrary to providing you with energy, is draining you and leaving you less focused. This is particularly true of calorie-rich foods. This is the reason why everyone wants to only sleep after the heavy Thanksgiving turkey meal.

If you think about it, there might be evolutionary reasons why fasting for some time makes people feel energetic and focused.

Human beings were not meant to always be in a full state because if you are always full, then you will never look for food. It was important to be in a fasted state because it is only in that state that hunger is felt. Hunger prompted the early man to go and look for food. So, it makes sense that it is only in the fasted state that the brain needs to be functioning at its best because it is in that state that they have to hunt for food. Hunting for food required a lot of energy and individuals who did not have the required energy obviously could not survive and compete.

Remember, it was always about the survival of the fittest. So, the early man had to be fit to survive and periods of fasting ensure that. Therefore, intermittent fasting will help you regain your energy and improve focus, which will increase your productivity no matter what your profession. is

Burn Fat

Last but not least, intermittent fasting will help you burn fat. Burning fat will help you become "fit" from "fat" and help you bid farewell to your love handles and overall flab. Blood samples were taken from people who were fasting for 12 – 24 hours. These people enter into a state called "ketosis." Ketosis is the state when the body turns to the extra fat stored, and fat burning happens. The more time the body is in ketosis state, the more fat is burned. Intermittent fasting is a very effective way to get into ketosis mode and boosting ketone levels.

Apart from fat burning, there is another significant effect of ketosis. It has shown to trigger the release of a molecule called BDNF, which provides strength to the neurons and brain connections linked to memory and learning. It is for this reason that some people experience clarity and work better with improved focus when they are fasting.

Intermittent fasting works as well as other diets floating around. The biggest benefit of intermittent fasting is that it provides a plethora of benefits with very minimal modifications to your life at zero cost. It is extremely cost effective since it does not prescribe special ingredients or fancy products, time-sensitive since no elaborate recipes are required. Unlike other diets, which may help you shed extra pounds and make you look good, intermittent fasting benefits the entire functioning of your body and mind. It significantly elevates your quality of life by improving all aspects of it with no extra effort.

This is the only method among the hundreds of diets that focus on a holistic approach rather than on quick-fix solutions that offer a temporary solution to your problems but do not do much in the long run. It can be tried easily wherever you are, and since it does not call for special recipes or ingredients, this can be easily practiced even when you are traveling either on work or on vacation.

The biggest area where most people cannot keep up with a diet is during holidays and travel. As most diets recommend specific recipes, specific ingredients and this can become cumbersome during holidays and especially when traveling. Many times, when you travel, you do not have access to a lot of stuff that is available at home, and this can deter you from following a diet. Another reason is that nobody wants to cook while traveling. Intermittent fasting lets you eat whatever is available as the only requirement is timing.

The fasting time is the only thing that you need to keep in mind while following intermittent fasting.

Time is in your hands. You have absolute control over the 24 hours available to you, and you can decide the fasting window based on your convenience.

So, in the next chapters, you will be introduced to the different methods of intermittent fasting, and you are free to choose whatever works for you based on your weight goals, lifestyle, work schedule, and dietary preferences. Almost all methods have shown results, and each has its benefits and disadvantages. Some call for extended periods of fasting and some moderate.

YOU choose who and what you want to be. Choose wisely.

Chapter Eight
Types of Intermittent Fasts and Best Practices to Follow While Fasting

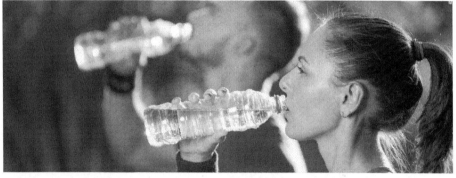

Fasts can be categorized in a variety of ways, however, the two criteria that are often used to segregate them, are:

What is allowed and not allowed?

As this book mainly deals with intermittent fasting, we will cover the various types and variations of intermittent fasting, however, before that let us have a close look at what practices should you follow while fasting.

In any regular fast, you have an eating period and a non-eating period. While you can eat various things in the eating period, you need to monitor what you eat in the non-eating period closely.

Drinks

Almost all fasts allow only noncaloric drinks in the non-eating or fasting phase. This includes drinks such as water, black tea, black coffee, green tea, etc. Additives like honey, sugar, fructose, agave nectar and all other forms of sugar should be avoided. In certain fasts artificial sweeteners such as aspartame, stevia and sucralose are allowed; however other varieties look down upon these as they contain chemicals that in turn are counterintuitive to the spirit of eating organic.

Water-only fast, as the name suggests allows only water to be consumed while fasting. Some variations allow practitioners to drink salt water.

Juice fast allows the consumption of juice along with water. Juice is a very subjective term and can mean a lot of things. Never drink packaged juices while fasting; these contain excessive amounts of sugars and preservatives that are harmful to the fast and for the body as well. Only drink freshly squeezed or pressed juices. Juices naturally contain sugars and calories, and therefore juice fasts are not true fasts. It is advised to avoid drinking a lot of fruit juices as they contain a high amount of sugar. Instead, try drinking green juice, i.e., juice of mixed vegetables such as spinach, kale, amaranth, etc. You can also add celery and a couple of slices of orange to the juice to make it tastier.

In a dry fast, no fluids are allowed, and you are supposed to follow a complete, strict fast. Muslims follow this kind of fast in the holy month of Ramadan. They avoid drinking any fluids while fasting. This sort of fast is extremely difficult to follow and may lead to dehydration as well.

All kinds of fasts will have some therapeutic benefits; however, you need to keep certain things in mind while fasting. Do not start a fast randomly, always conduct research and choose a plan that suits your needs and lifestyle.

Let us have a look at common drinks that you can consume while fasting.

Water

You must consume lots of water if you want to fast successfully. Water will keep you hydrated and will keep you full for a long time. Try to drink at least two liters of water every day. If you do not like drinking plain water, squeeze a slice of lemon in it. You can also make cucumber infused water. Avoid adding artificial flavors as they can prove to be counterproductive.

Tea

All types of teas can be consumed while fasting including oolong, black, green, herbal, etc. You can also blend different teas for added taste. Do not add any cream, milk, sugar or sweetener to the tea. While all teas are good, green tea should be the beverage of your choice. Green tea contains high amounts of catechins that act as appetite suppressors.

If you dislike plain tea, add spices such as nutmeg, cinnamon or cardamom to enhance the taste and flavor of the tea. People who like spicy tea can also add crushed peppercorn to their brew.

Herbal teas are not true teas as they lack tealeaves. While not true teas, herbal teas can help you with your fasts. Ginger tea, mint tea, chamomile tea, cinnamon tea, lavender tea, etc. All have appetite suppressing properties. As herbal teas do not contain caffeine, you can have them any time of the day.

Coffee

You can have both caffeinated and decaf coffee on a fast. Do not add cream or sugar to your coffee. You can add spices to make it tastier. You can also have iced coffee; however, do not add sugar or any other sweetener to it.

Bone Broth

If you eat meat, you can have bone broth while fasting. Bone broth is made of bones of fish, beef, chicken, lamb, pork and other animals. To make bone broth, add bones, a few vegetables, and seasoning to a large pot of water and let it simmer for 8-30 hours. While bone broth contains more nutrients if you do not eat meat you can make vegetable broth as well. Do not add bouillon cubes to the broth. Do not buy canned broth as they often contain artificial flavors.

Add sea salt to your broth to make it tastier. Sea salt will also help you to conquer dehydration and salt deficiency. Do not replace sea salt with other salts as sea salt contains traces of other minerals including magnesium and potassium. These minerals are good during fasting.

Chapter Nine
Types of Intermittent Fast

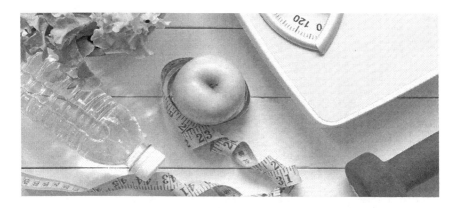

While many types of fasts exist, the most commonly followed fast for weight loss is intermittent fast. Even intermittent fast can be divided into a variety of types. In this section let us have a look some of the most commonly followed types of intermittent fasts. All of them are devised according to the needs and requirements of various users. Go through them and check out which one of them is the most suitable for you.

16/8 Method

One of the most popular forms of intermittent fasting is the 16/8 intermittent fast. In this fast, you are allowed to eat foods in a set window of 8 hours and are supposed to abstain from food for 16 hours. Repeating this forms a cycle, which can be done as per your personal preference. You can perform the fast twice a week, once a week or even every day. 16/8 fast has become extremely popular in recent times as it allows people to lose weight and burn fat quickly and healthily. 16/8 diet does not have any strict rules, and you can get results without a lot of effort. Along with weight loss, 16/8 fast can help you improve your blood sugar levels and can also boost the functioning of your brain.

Starting intermittent fast is simple, sustainable and safe. To begin, pick a window of 8 hours to eat whatever you want in that window (in proper portions). That's it. This window can be adjusted according to the needs of the practitioner. For instance, some people like to have two meals per day, so they tend to choose a noon window, i.e., their eating window starts at noon and ends around 8 PM. This allows them to have lunch and dinner. As sleeping hours are counted in the fasting window, you need to stay hungry until lunch on the next day, and you will effectively complete a day of 16/8 fast. So basically, 16/8 fast can be as easy as skipping your breakfast and eating your dinner early every day.

For people who do not like skipping breakfast can choose a morning window where it starts around 9 AM and ends around 5 PM. In this option, you can have three meals in a day however you will have to either eat dinner before 5 PM or have a light snack around that time.

It solely depends on your needs and the time frame that suits you. You can divide your meals according to your schedule. For instance, you may consume three meals in your 8-hour window or can have many small meals throughout the eating period. Eating small meals throughout the window will keep your blood sugar levels stable and will also keep you full for a long time.

While you can eat anything you want in your eating window, it is recommended to eat nutritious and low-calorie foods and beverages. This will keep your calories under control ensuring weight loss.

Ideally, your meals should include fruit like bananas, apples, oranges, peaches, berries, pears, etc. This should be accompanied with various grains like rice, quinoa, oats, buckwheat, etc. You should also consume poultry, meat, olive oil, nuts, eggs, etc. to ensure an ample supply of proteins and fats.
Along with the above food products, you can consume various unsweetened beverages such as black tea, water, coffee, green tea, etc. These will keep you satiated for a long time and will also

prevent dehydration. Remember, you must consume proper, nutritional meals while following the 16/8 fast or else it may lead to a variety of problems.

Problems with 16/8 fast

While 16/8 fast is one of the most popular forms of intermittent fasting, it does have specific problems and drawbacks that you need to take into account before beginning it. One of the biggest problems that people may face while following the 16/8 fast is overeating. Some people may try to overcompensate by eating heavy meals. 16/8 intermittent fasting may cause certain other short-term negative side effects such as hunger, fatigue, weakness, etc. But these routines will subside as soon as you become habitual of it.

5:2 Diet

5:2 diet is another very popular form of intermittent fasting. As the name suggests, in this diet you can eat for five days while you need to restrict your calories for the remaining two days. This diet is also known as Fast Diet, which was popularized by Michael Mosley, a famous British journalist and doctor. The calorie restriction depends on various factors including gender, lifestyle and health of the practitioner, however; women should restrict their calories to 500 while men around 700.

Why does this diet work? According to practitioners, you will feel hungry on the fasting days; however, you will continue to fast as you will know that the next day is the day of the feast. Therefore, with little self-control, you will be able to follow this date with ease.

If you are into endurance training, it is advised to avoid this diet. If you still want to follow it, you should consult with a dietician and devise a plan according to your requirements.

Here is a sample plan from Mosley that you can follow while performing this fast.

Day 1
Breakfast:
Oats Porridge (40g) - 255 Calories
Dinner:
Beetroot with feta salad - 125 calories
Snack:
Sliced apples- 145 calories
Total calorie count: 525

Day 2
Breakfast:
Sweet plums with sugarless yogurt - 145 calories
Dinner:
Crackers with slices of tuna - 253 calories
Snack:
Miso soup - 32 calories
Total calorie count: 430

Day 3
Breakfast:
Soft boiled egg with asparagus sticks - 90 calories
Dinner:
Turkey burgers and corn-on-the-cob - 328 calories
(Do not add bread)
Snack:
Frozen grapes - 60 calories
Total calorie count: 478 calories

Day 4
Breakfast:
Muesli - 228 calories
Dinner:
Roasted vegetables - 261 calories
Snack:
Sugar-free jelly - 4 calories
Total calorie count: 495

Day 5
Breakfast:
Spinach omelet - 160 calorie
Dinner:
Hummus and crudités - 175 calories
Snack:
Edamame beans (60g) - 84 calories
Total calorie count: 419

Day 6
Breakfast:
Banana with low-fat yogurt - 177 calories
Dinner:
Turkey breasts and spinach - 216 calories
Snack:
A small cup of Popcorn - 59 calories
Total calorie count: 452

Day 7
Breakfast:
Apple, ginger and celery smoothie - 107 calories
Dinner:
Pitta pizza - 178 calories
Snack:
One small cup blueberries with a few almonds - 137 calories
Total calorie count: 422

Day 8
Breakfast:
Mixed berries - 115 calories
Dinner:
Harissa chicken and vegetable couscous - 314 calories
Snack:
a handful of Pistachios - 60 calories
Total calorie count - 489 calories

Day 9
Breakfast:
Blueberry Buttermilk Pancakes (2) - 206 calories
Dinner:
Roasted red pepper with tomato soup - 128 calories
Snack:
One small cup pumpkin and sunflower seeds - 90 calories
Total calorie count: 424 calories

Day 10

Breakfast:
Fruit muesli (50g) - 190 calories
Dinner:
Pesto salmon - 293 calories
Snack:
A small cup of cherries - 23 calories
Total calorie count: 506 calories

You can adjust these meal plans according to your needs and tastes. For instance, if you do not like eating fish, you can replace it with anything that has similar calories.

24 hour Fast

24 hour fast, as the name suggests is fasting for 24 hours once or twice a week. This method was made popular by Brad Pilon and has become extremely popular in recent times.

The plan of this diet is quite easy, however following it may prove to be quite difficult to many. A common plan of this diet includes eating dinner today and then avoid all meals until the dinner the next day. This means you will fast for 24 hours in all. Some people do it lunch to lunch.

This method works wonders for people who want to lose weight, as it is extremely difficult to eat calories worth an entire day in one sitting. While the plan is effective, it is difficult to follow. Not many people can stick to it. Certain people feel nausea, weakness, brain fog, etc. in this fast.

Only solid food is allowed while performing this fast. You may, however, consume non-caloric beverages and water. If you plan to do this fast to lose weight, then it is advised to consume healthy and low-calorie food on your eating days.

As said earlier, it is quite difficult to follow 24 hours fast so it is recommended to start slow. You may start with a 14-16 hour diet and then slowly advance towards a complete, 24 hours fast. This will allow your body to become accustomed to the fast gradually which may make the overall ordeal less cumbersome.

While nutrition is the major reason why we eat food, it is not the only one. We also eat food according to our mood and atmosphere. For instance, some people eat a lot when they are sad or elated. We often eat according to our emotions. It is, therefore, necessary to understand that there exist two kinds of hunger and how they are different than each other. If you understand the difference between the two, you will be able to eat accordingly.

One of the best ways to understand the difference between the two hungers is by doing the 24 hours fast. This fast allows you to understand the difference between emotional hunger and physiological hunger. Let us have a look at both of these, one by one.

Physiological hunger

You experience physiological hunger when your body, brain, and muscles are tired or are in a low-energy state. People often experience this kind of hunger after a particularly demanding workout. You also experience this sort of hunger when you exert yourself physically or mentally. Physiological hunger is a signal from your brain, which means that your energy has gone down and it needs to be replenished. When you feel physiological hunger you should consume fats, carbohydrates and fats. This will provide energy to help your tissues grow.

Emotional Hunger

Emotional hunger is quite different as compared to physiological hunger. This is a type of hunger that you feel when a situation, for instance, your emotions or your mood make you eat something. While physiological hunger creates a hunger of need, emotional hunger creates a hunger of desire. Emotional hunger is much stronger than physiological hunger; however physiological hunger is far more important for health and wellbeing.

It is necessary to understand the difference between these two as they play a huge role in your health and fitness. A 24-hour fast is an extremely difficult feat to pull off; however, it will allow you to enjoy true independence from food, at least for a small amount of time.

While intermittent fasting does not guarantee instant results, you can still feel the difference in your body and mind after one 24 hours fast. These results get amplified over time and therefore, the more you fast, the more results you will get. As intermittent fasting is not a fad diet, these results, though slow, will not go away.

Let us have a look at a 24-hour fast plan that you can incorporate in your schedule.

24-hour fast plan (weekly)

As the name suggests, this is a 24-hour fast plan that you perform on any one-day of the week. This day is supposed to be according to your needs; however, it is recommended to choose a day on which you will be largely sedentary. Ideally, people tend to choose a weekday instead of Sunday, as weekends can be hectic. If you are ready to sacrifice your social life, then Sunday is the best choice for doing a 24 hour fast.

Let us assume you decide to fast on Sunday. Ideally, your schedule should go like this.

Steps

1. **8 PM Saturday**
   Eat your dinner and drink lots of water.
2. **9 PM Saturday**
   Begin your fast.
3. **11 PM Saturday**
   Go to sleep.
4. **8 AM Sunday**
   Drink lots of water. You may also have 2-3 cups of freshly brewed green tea.
5. **12 PM Sunday**
   Drink lots of water. You may also have 2-3 cups of freshly brewed green tea.
6. **3 PM Sunday**

Drink lots of water. You may also have 2-3 cups of freshly brewed green tea.

7. **8 PM Sunday**

   End your fast by consuming an apple.

8. **9 PM Sunday**

   Have a small dinner with low carb foods along with lean protein. Drink lots of water.

9. **8 AM Monday**

   Resume your regular eating schedule.

What to 'eat' while fasting?

While consuming anything substantial while fasting is prohibited, you may consume lots of non-caloric drinks instead. These include:

Water

You should consume 2-3 cups of water whenever you are advised to drink water. This will confuse your gut and will make you full. It will also curb your cravings.

Green tea

Instead of water, you can also drink 2-3 cups of freshly brewed green tea.
Green tea contains hunger-suppressing elements that also curb your cravings.
If you ever feel hungry, have a couple of cups of green tea.

Strategies to follow while doing the 24 hours fast:

Use Green Tea:

While green tea is not essential to fasting, it can make the overall process easier. Green tea can suppress appetite and curb the feeling of hunger.

Understand your body cues:

The human body is a complex machine, and it gives out signals of stress, pleasure, trouble, etc. to make you aware of its condition. Be aware and try to look out for these signals. If you feel too stressed or upset while fasting, relax and try to understand the nature of your hunger. Keep healthy food items at hand when you break your fast. Hunger can turn people, and if you don't have healthy food items handy, it is possible that you will end up consuming high-calorie foods. Don't let hunger turn into hanger.

Stocking healthy food in your pantry will ensure that you do not binge on unhealthy snacks when your fast ends.

Modified 24 Hour Fast

While 24 hour fast can lead to a lot of benefits, it should be noted that not everyone could do it. Doing a 24 hour fast is quite difficult. The difficulty is severe for people who have diabetes as long fasts can lead to hypoglycemia. If you feel that you can get hypoglycemic, always keep food handy. This will prevent any unfortunate and unseen accidents.

While 'hanger' is not a real, severe issue, excess hunger can make you hungry. If you cannot stay hungry for a long time, try to begin with shorter fasts and increase the length of your fasts gradually.

If you find it excessively difficult to follow a regular 24 hours fast, you may follow a modified fast. People who belong to one or more categories mentioned below should also follow a modified version of the 24 hours fast.

Categories

- Type 1 Diabetes Patients
- Type 2 Diabetes Patients
- People suffering from prediabetes
- You have low blood sugar
- You can hangry easily
- Fasting makes you violent
- Fasting makes you unpleasant

Hypoglycemia

Hypoglycemia is the primary cause why the 24-hour fast is difficult. When you don't consume any calories for a long time, your brain may feel starved which may lead to a variety of symptoms. Some of these symptoms are given below.

- Mood swings
- Frustration

- Inability to concentrate
- Anger
- Shaky hands
- Slurred speech
- Excessive Sweating

The Difference between true and modified 24 hours fast

The biggest difference between modified and regular or true 24 hour fast is that you can consume some amount of calories on modified fast. You can eat around 100-150 calories per meal. While modified 24 hours fast is not as good as a true 24 hours fast, it is still extremely beneficial. It will also reduce any side effects of the 24 hours fast.

Let us assume you decide to fast on Sunday. Ideally, your schedule should go like this.

Steps

1. **8 PM Saturday**
   Eat your dinner and drink lots of water.

2. **9 PM Saturday**
   Begin your fast.

3. **11 PM Saturday**
   Go to sleep.

4. **8 AM Sunday**
   Drink lots of water and one small bowl of vegetable soup.

5. **12 PM Sunday**
   Drink lots of water. You may also have 2-3 cups of freshly brewed green tea.

6. **3 PM Sunday**

   Drink lots of water. Have a small bowl of vegetable soup or consume a couple of slices of a fruit of your choice.

7. **8 PM Sunday**

   End your fast by consuming an apple.

8. **9 PM Sunday**

   Have a small dinner with low carb foods along with lean protein. Drink lots of water.

9. **8 AM Monday**

   Resume your normal eating schedule.

100-200 Calorie Meal Options

1 Cup of Vegetable Soup
Your soup should contain celery, beets, carrots, cucumbers, kale, spinach, tomatoes, etc. Do not eat more than 8 oz. of soup. You can eat 1-2 pieces of your favorite fruit

Eat 1-2 piece of fruit
You can have any fruit however apples and oranges are preferred. Avoid mango, as it is a calorie-rich fruit.

Vegetable soup can be replaced with the following things as well:

1-2 Servings of Vegetables
Simple broiled or steam vegetables such as tomatoes, cauliflowers, okra, etc.
can be consumed instead of vegetable soup. Do not add excess seasoning.
One-tablespoon nuts You may consume a small number of nuts such as almonds, cashews, etc.

Salad

A small serving of salad containing cabbage, lettuce, spinach, etc. can be consumed instead of vegetable soup.

Negative Energy balance

Negative energy balance is a condition when your rate of energy expenditure becomes higher than your rate of energy consumption. This means you will continue to lose energy throughout your fast.

While many people think that they will consume twice the amount of food right after they finish their fast, however, this is easier said than done. It is difficult to consume a lot of food at one go which means the negative energy balance will continue even after your fasting period is over.

Negative energy balance is one of the biggest assets of intermittent fasting and especially 24-hour fasting. Other diets recommend calorie restriction in which you continue to feel hungry and irritable almost every day, whereas in 24 hours fast, you fast only once a week, this allows you to be happy and satiated on the rest of the days. Intermittent fasting will not hinder your mental and physical wellbeing in any way.

A 24-hour fast is a great way to find the differences and balance between emotional and physiological hunger. It is a great way of losing weight and improving your overall health. It can also help you to improve your cardiovascular health.

While fasting may seem quite difficult in the beginning, once you begin it you will realize that it is not that difficult. This feeling will grow steadily when you start observing results.

Alternate-Day Fasting

In this type of intermittent fasting, you are supposed to fast one day and then feast the next. On the day of fast, you are allowed around 500 calories. This version is supposed to be beneficial for your health. It is also easy to follow as compared to other forms of fasting. However, it is not meant for beginners, as it will leave you feeling hungry for 3-4 days a week.

Here is a short meal plan that you can follow to make fasting easy.

Soups and Salads

As said earlier, you are supposed to consume around 500-700 calories per day according to your health, gender, and body structure. You can consume a no-sodium tomato soup topped with greens or with a side of greens along with skinless chicken dressed with lemon juice on your fasting day. This can be followed with some fresh fruit such as strawberries, orange, melon, etc. Avoid eating mango and similar fruit as they contain high amounts of calories. This plan is suitable for women. Men may increase the quantity slightly to meet their calorie requirements.

Lean Beef

You can eat beef while doing the alternate fast diet. Avoid picking greasy or fatty cuts of meat instead pick lean cuts like sirloin or tenderloin. Do not eat high-calorie side dishes with the steak. Women may consume a medium sized seared steak with caramelized onions and some cheese. This can be paired with sautéed chard and polenta. Again men may either increase the quantity of the described items or may include other food items to meet their calorific demand. Simple and healthy vegetables like asparagus can be added to the diet to make it healthier.

Seafood

Seafood is necessary while fasting as it ensures an adequate amount of omega-3 fatty acids. These acids are essential for the proper functioning of the heart. Women can eat shrimp served with sautéed garlic and onion, along with fresh tomatoes. Later they may eat a tortilla with chopped avocado and brown rice. Men can increase the calories by adding sautéed kale and other greens to the above-mentioned plan.

Avoid Meat

If you want to skip meat on a particular day or you don't eat meat, then you can still follow alternate fast.

For a meatless fast option, women can eat a whole-wheat pizza topped with simple vegetables and some mozzarella. This should be followed with some vegetable soup and vegetable salad. If you consume dairy, you may add yogurt as well. Men may add a ripe apple to their diet to fulfill their quota of calories.

The Warrior Diet

The warrior diet has become extremely popular in recent times. It is also a type of intermittent fasting. In this fast, you are supposed to consume foods in short windows. This diet is supposed to provide you with mental clarity and can help you lose weight as well. Let us have a close look at the warrior diet in this section.

What Is the Warrior Diet?

Ori Hofmekler, an ex-member of the Israeli Special Forces is credited with the creation of this diet. He transitioned to the field of nutrition after his stint with the Special Forces and created this diet in 2001.

The warrior diet comes under the umbrella term of intermittent fasting. It is based on the dietary patterns of the ancient warriors who used to consume very little food during the day and then had feasts at night. According to Hofmekler, this diet has been designed in such a way that it can improve the way we feel, eat, look and perform. Therefore it is a diet that leads to the overall development of mind and the body. Hofmekler did not use any scientific basis for this diet; rather he used his observations and beliefs to do so. In this diet, people tend to under eat for about 20 hours a day and then eat their desired food around night.

In the 20 hours phase, dieters are allowed to eat small amounts of boiled eggs, dairy products, fruit and vegetables, etc. Dieters are also allowed to drink non-calorie fluids and drinks such as black tea, coffee, green tea, etc. After this period is over, dieters can consume anything they want in a small, 4-hour eating window. While you are allowed to eat anything you want in this window, it is advised to eat organic and healthy foods. This will ensure that you healthily lose weight.

To get started, it is recommended to follow a three-week plan in the beginning. This plan then can be continued to a full-fledged warrior diet.

Problems of Warrior Diet

While the warrior diet has a lot of benefits, it does have some problems that can be a deal breaker for many.

Difficulty

One of the biggest problems with the warrior diet is that it is difficult. It is difficult to stay hungry throughout the day. This is especially difficult to do while socializing and performing your day-to-day activities. If your job is not sedentary, then the warrior diet may seem almost impossible to you. This diet is not ideal for the lifestyle of a lot of people.

Unsuitable for Many

The warrior diet is unsuitable for many people. Like other forms of intermittent fasting the following people should not follow it:

- Athletes
- People with eating disorders
- Children
- Pregnant women
- Nursing women
- Underweight or malnourished people

Eating Disorder

In this diet, you are supposed to overeat. This may prove to be counter-reactive for a lot of people. While Hofmekler argues that one should stop eating when one feels full, not all people can follow this. The warrior diet may lead to harmful binging and food addiction in certain people if not done properly.

Side Effects

The warrior diet may cause certain side effects including:

- Dizziness
- Fatigue
- Low energy
- Anxiety
- Lightheadedness
- Extreme Hunger
- Insomnia
- Constipation
- Hypoglycemia
- Hormonal imbalance
- Fainting
- Weight Gain
- Irritability

With these certain health professionals are of the opinion that the warrior diet may not provide practitioners with ample nutrients, however, this problem can be solved by having multivitamins regularly.

The above problems can be solved by consuming calorie-rich, nutrient-rich foods throughout the day. For this, you need to make a proper schedule and a diet plan.

Plans

As said earlier, Hofmekler recommends dieters to follow an initial 3-week plan before moving on to a more severe warrior diet. This plan is divided into three phases. Let us have a look at them one by one.

Phase I
Week 1: Detox

In this first phase, you are supposed to get rid of all the toxins present in your body. This process will prepare your body and mind for the next phases.

To begin, start under eating and continue to under eat for 20 hours during the day. You may eat dairy, vegetable juices, hard-boiled eggs, clear broth, raw veggies and fruit in this phase.

You may consume coffee, tea, water, etc. with small servings of milk throughout the day.

Phase II
Week 2: High Fat Phase

Once again to begin, start under eating and continue to under eat for 20 hours during the day. You may eat dairy, vegetable juices, hard-boiled eggs, clear broth, raw veggies and fruit in this phase.

Once the fasting period is over, you may eat small amounts of cheese, cooked vegetables, lean animal proteins, salads with oil and vinegar dressing and one handful of nuts, etc. Eat the nuts, as your body needs a lot of healthy fats in this phase. Do not consume any starch of grains in this phase.

Phase III
Week Three: Last Phase

In this phase, you are supposed to cycle between high protein and high carb intake.

For instance

- Monday, Tuesday - High Carbs

- Wednesday - High Protein
- Thursday - High Carbs
- Friday, Saturday - High Proteins
- Sunday - High carbs

On high-carb days you may consume:
Once again to begin, start under eating and continue to under eat for 20 hours during the day. You may eat dairy, vegetable juices, hard-boiled eggs, clear broth, raw veggies and fruit in this phase.

Once the fasting period is over, you may eat small amounts of cheese, cooked vegetables, lean animal proteins, salads with oil and vinegar dressing. Along with the above foods consume at least one of the following carbs - potatoes, corn, pasta, oats, barley etc.

On high-protein, low-carb days you can eat:
Once again to begin, start under eating and continue to under eat for 20 hours during the day. You may eat dairy, vegetable juices, hard-boiled eggs, clear broth, raw veggies and fruit in this phase.

Once the fasting period is over, you may eat small amounts of cheese, cooked vegetables, lean animal proteins, salads with oil and vinegar dressing and sides of freshly cooked vegetables.

Once all the three phases are over, Hofmekler recommends starting from phase one again. It is also possible to avoid going through the complete cycle, and you may continue to follow the steps given under the under the eating section for 20 hours followed by steps given in the overeating phase.

There are no set calorie restrictions or portion sizes in the warrior diet. It is recommended to have multivitamins and other supplements while following this diet. You may consult your dietician or GP to find out which supplements you need.

It is recommended to incorporate some form of exercise in your dietary regime. You may perform speed training or cardio. This will promote fat loss.

What to eat and what not to eat

Dieters can eat everything including whole grains, unprocessed foods, fruit, etc. But they should avoid processed foods, sugars, sweeteners, preservatives, etc. Do not eat products with chemicals and artificial coloring as they contain harmful toxins.

Foods to eat in small portions in the less eating phase:

- Fruit: Apples, bananas, mango, kiwi, pineapple, peach, etc.
- Vegetable juices: Carrot, beet, celery, etc.
- Raw vegetables: Peppers, Greens, carrots, mushrooms, onions, etc.
- Broth: Beef, Chicken, etc.
- Condiments: Olive oil, apple cider vinegar, etc.
- Dairy: Milk, yogurt, cottage cheese, etc.
- Protein: Hard-boiled or poached eggs
- Beverages: Water, seltzer, coffee, tea, etc.

Foods to Eat In the Overeating Phase:

- Steamed/ Boiled/ Broiled vegetables: Cauliflower, zucchini, Brussels sprouts, greens, etc.
- Proteins: Chicken, fish, steak, turkey, eggs, etc.
- Starches: Beans, corn, potatoes, sweet potatoes, etc.
- Grains: Oats, pasta, quinoa, whole-grain bread, barley, etc.
- Dairy: Milk, yogurt, cheese, etc.
- Fats: Nuts, olive oil, etc.

Foods You Should Avoid:

- Cookies and cakes
- Candy
- Chips
- Processed carbohydrates
- Fried Foods

- Fast food
- Processed meats (lunch meats, bacon)
- Artificial sweeteners

Erratic or Spontaneous Fast:

Spontaneous fast or erratic fast does not have any structure, and it is randomized fasting. You do not need any preplanning to follow this fast that makes it suitable for people with hectic schedules. While this fast does not have as many benefits as 24 hours fast, but it is better than other forms of diet.

One of the easiest ways to do this fast is skipping meals whenever you can. If you don't feel hungry, do not eat anything. You will be surprised to find how eating can become a habit. Many times we eat just because its time to eat, I.e., our body gets conditioned to eat at a particular time. When this time arrives, our brain sends a signal to eat. This signal is sent even if we are not hungry.

Don't worry; if you do not eat for a few hours, you will not hit the starvation mode. You won't lose muscles either. Our bodies have evolved in such a way that we can handle long periods of starvation without losing the structure of integrity of our bodies. So if you do not feel hungry, skip that meal and eat at the next meal instead. Similarly, if you are traveling and do not feel like eating have a short fast instead. Skipping meals whenever you can is spontaneous fasting.

Whenever you are not fasting, try to eat healthy foods. This will ensure your weight loss. Intermittent fasting is not for everyone. It is not something that anyone needs to do. It is just another tool in the toolbox that can be useful for some people.

Intermittent fasting is not meant for everyone. Some people think that anyone can do it. But in the end, remember, whichever diet you follow - always eat healthily.

Chapter Ten
Myths about Intermittent Fasting

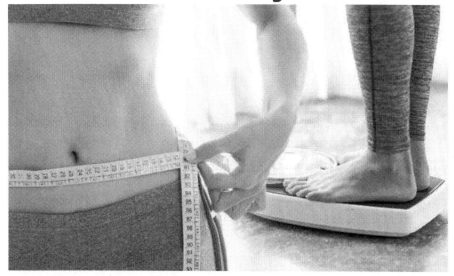

As explained in the last chapter, fasting is one of the oldest methods of weight loss, yet it should not come as a surprise that not many people believe fasting to be a real diet. Not many are aware of the multitude of benefits that a person can get if they fast regularly. Many myths are prevalent in society about fasting. This chapter will focus on these myths and will try to disapprove them one by one.

Some of the most common myths associated with fasting include:

- Fasting is not suitable for athletes and people who want to put on muscles.

- Fasting can lead to low blood sugar.

- Fasting will make you starve or will induce 'starvation mode'.

- Fasting is bad because you will end up eating more calories than regular in your eating period.

- Fasting is not healthy because you do not get adequate and enough nutrients.

- Fasting is a fad diet or is some ancient hogwash that has no place in the modern world.

Almost all of the above myths have already been proven false by research and scientists, but like a stain that won't go these myths continue to plague the mindset of society. A large chunk of the population still thinks that fasting will make them waste away or that it will prove detrimental to their fitness and health. This cannot be farther away from the truth. Fasting has numerous health benefits, and all of them have been approved by science. All these benefits will be discussed in depth in the next chapters but first, let us have a look at the myths of fasting.

Fasting induces 'starvation mode'

There is a myth doing rounds that fasting leads to 'starvation mode.' Before debunking this myth, let us have a look at what starvation mode is.

Why do people think it is bad to skip meals? Let us assume that a healthy, regular person eats three meals per day. In one year this person will have consumed over one thousand meals. If you take away one meal per day from this huge number, it is absurd to think that it will cause any significant damage.

Starvation mode can be defined as a state in which the body shuts down certain functions which slows down metabolism severely. A slowed metabolism works against weight loss, and it may even increase your weight. This effect can be studied by looking BMR or basal metabolic rate. BMR measures the amount of energy that our body uses to function. This includes the energy required for the brain and various other bodily functions to work properly. The food you consume every day provides your body with calories, which are then burned to perform these functions. Extra calories can be burned by exercising regularly.

BMR is not a fixed number, and it fluctuates according to your body and the surrounding. For instance, some people become extremely sensitive to temperature drops after a certain age. Our body uses calories to keep itself warm in the winter. High metabolism rate allows for proper heat distribution; however, metabolism often slows down with age, which makes people more sensitive to cold.

It has been observed that a drastic reduction in calorie consumption can lead to low BMR. For instance, if your regular calorie intake for a day is 2500 and you bring it down to 1500, it is possible that your BMR will go down by 30 percent. In contrast, if you start eating more, your BMR will grow as well.

Low BMR makes you tired, cold, less energetic and hungry. You will feel lethargic all the time. Your body essentially tries to function properly by conserving energy. Reduced metabolism is extremely harmful to people who want to lose weight. It makes you feel lethargic and uneasy. Even if you manage to lose weight on a reduced BMR, it is bound to come back. This is why many fad diets such as juice cleanse, which leaves you feeling tired and hungry, and their results do not last for a long time.

When you drastically reduce your calorie consumption for a long duration, your body thinks that you are starving and it goes into starvation mode. It reduces your BMR and tries to conserve as much energy as possible. When you fast, your calories get restricted as well, which is why many people believe that it can lead to starvation mode as well.

That fasting leads to starvation mode is a myth. Short-term fasting does not lead to starvation or decrease in BMR. If this were the case, then humans would not have survived. During the long and cold winter in the Stone Age, our hunting fathers must have gone days together without food. Many of them probably died of starvation; however, as human species is still thriving, then it can be assumed that the stronger ones survived. As we are the progeny of survivors, we too can survive short-term fasts.

In contrast to the myth, our metabolism goes up while fasting. When we fast, or when our food intake becomes zero, our body starts to look for materials other than food to burn to get energy. As our body is a complex machine, it keeps excess energy stored in the form of fats. While fasting, our body turns to these stores of fats for energy. As our body consumes more 'food' in the form of fats, it receives high amounts of energy, which it tries to spend. This expenditure is in the form of increased BMR.

The above phenomenon has been proved by a variety of experiment.
Following are two of such experiments:

In one study a group of random subjects was asked to fast for twenty-two days where it was found that the BMR of these subjects had not gone down at all. These subjects did not go into starvation mode; instead, their fat burning rate went up by 58%, and their bodies had started switching over to burning fat. They did not feel lethargic or tired and instead felt energized.

In the second study, it was observed that BMR went up by 12% after four days of continuous fasting. The levels of noradrenaline went up by 117%, and the body switched over from burning food to burning stored fats for energy. Noradrenaline is an essential hormone that keeps our body ready for action; in other words, it keeps us energized.

So where did 'fasting is unhealthy' myth come from? It is assumed that this myth started with the market encouraging consumers to buy food. Each year corporations spend thousands of dollars on advertising so that consumers will buy their products. Certain snacks bar that portrays hungry people to be grouchy is a classic example of such advertisements. But, as proven above, this is just a myth.

Fasting is not suitable for people who want to put on muscles.

Another myth that is very commonly associated with fasting is that it eats up muscles. According to this myth, our body will start burning muscles for energy if it is starved.

While our body starts using muscles as a source of energy, mere short-term fasting cannot trigger this reaction. Our body stores excess energy in the form of fats and uses these stores when no other source of energy is available. Similarly, the body does not use muscles as a source of energy until the fat stores deplete significantly. This happens only when the levels of body fats go under 4%. All mammals have this property as it ensures our survival.

The concern over muscle-loss is grossly misplaced. Fasting only decreases fat stores and body weight, not muscle mass.

Our body uses three major nutrients to provide us energy viz — proteins, fats and carbohydrates or carbs. When we fast, our body starts using carbohydrates as a source of energy in the beginning. Once the body runs out of carbs to burn it switches over to fats. While fat burning increases, carb burning slowly decreases and stops at zero. Similarly, protein burning starts going down as well. Therefore, while fasting, instead of burning muscles our body tries to conserve them.

Basically, why would our body spend so much time and energy in storing fats if it meant to chow down on proteins as soon as we start fasting? Muscles are not meant to store energy. Muscle gain and loss normally is a function of exercise. You can't expect to put on muscles with dietary changes only; you must exercise. While supplements can help with muscle gain, mere supplements will not give you gains. If you still believe that fasting may induce muscle loss, you may increase the intensity or frequency of your workout. This will ensure the shape and size of your muscles.

Fasting can lead to low blood sugar.

Proper and regular blood sugar levels are necessary for the normal functioning of our body. Low blood sugar can lead to a variety of problems right from feeling sweaty and shaky to other serious disorders. Many people believe that fasting can lower your blood sugar levels drastically, but this does not happen. While starvation can lead to lower blood sugar levels, mere fasting won't. Our body breaks glycogen while fasting to create glucose. This is a daily process, and our body does it while we sleep.

People who fast for spiritual or religious reasons often proclaim that fasting makes them more active and clear-headed. Some people have also proclaimed that it made them feel euphoric. 'Spiritual fasters' often believe this effect to be some spiritual enlightenment. The scientific reason behind this feeling is ketones. Ketones make us euphoric and active. They make us clear headed.

When you fast for more than twenty-four hours, our body starts using glycogen stores and they soon deplete. The liver then starts to manufacture new glucose with the help of gluconeogenesis. This process uses glycerol, which in turn is a byproduct of the fat burning process. This means that you do not need to consume glucose to maintain glucose levels while fasting for short-term, i.e., intermittent fasting.

Another myth related to sugar depletion is that the brain only uses glucose for energy. The human brain can also use ketone particles as a source of energy. This function is triggered when our body does not have ample food available. Therefore, when glucose is not available, the body starts burning fats to produce ketones for energy.

Fasting can lead to Overeating

People often tend to think that fasting for a certain period may lead to compensatory overeating. Missing even a single meal can make you hungrier which will lead you to eat more than you eat regularly. This will prove to be counter-intuitive to your goal of losing weight.

According to certain recent studies, this myth is half-true. According to these studies, there is a slight growth of calorie intake on the first day of fasting. But you need to take into account that you will be skipping a meal, so even if you overeat in the beginning, at the end of the day, you will still end up with a deficit.

While you may consume more calories, in the beginning, repeated fasting will counter this effect. According to the personal experiences of many people who fast regularly, once fasting becomes a habit, your hunger subsides as well, and you do not feel hungry for a long time.

Fasting and Nutrients

When a person fasts, they skip certain meals of the day. This has led to the propagation of a myth that people who fast regularly do not get enough nutrients from their diet. Before moving on to debunk this myth let us have a look at what nutrients are.

Nutrients are the substances that we gain from food that are essential for us to survive. There are two kinds of nutrients — macronutrients and micronutrients. Micronutrients include minerals and vitamins while macronutrients include fats, proteins and carbohydrates.

Micronutrient deficiency is often seen in developing and underdeveloped nations and is rarely observed in the developed world. Short-term fasting does not affect micronutrient intake at all, however, if you want to perform a longer fast, I.e., fast that is longer than a day, it is advised to take a multivitamin tablet. Any simple multivitamin will take care of any scare of deficiency.

Macronutrient deficiency too is quite rare in developed nations. As our body does not need any specific form of carbohydrates for functioning, it is almost impossible to become carb deficient. It is possible to get protein and fat deficiency. If we do not get certain essential amino acids and fatty acids our body cannot function properly. The body normally gains most of these from our day-to-day diet and loses them in stool and urine. When you fast, your bowel movements decrease. Here, the body starts conserving proteins and fats and tries to recycle them instead of excreting them.

While our body tries hard to compensate for fats and proteins, it is still a good choice to go on a low carb diet after fasting. This will replenish your stores of fats and proteins.

It has been advised that children, pregnant women and lactating women should avoid fasting as these people require more nutrients than regular adults.

Fasting doesn't work & it's a gimmick

The people who believe fasting is fake are the same people who did not believe Yoga when it was first adopted in the western world. Fasting has a scientific base, and it is impossible to deny this. Fasting will help you lose weight.

Chapter Eleven
Tips and FAQs of Fasting

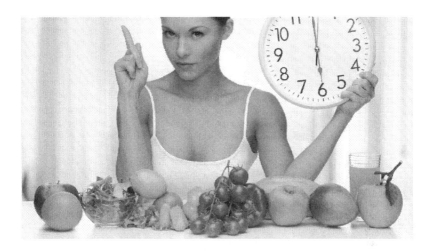

Fasting was an integral part of many religions and cultures once upon a time. It still is a part of the normal life of many religions throughout the world, including Muslims, Orthodox, Hinduism, Jainism, etc. In these examples, fasting is a communal practice as you are fasting with your friends and family. This allows you to have peer support, which ensures the success of your fast. However, when you plan to perform a fast alone, you have no peer support that makes it difficult to stick to one. This chapter will try to cover important advice and FAQs that will help you perform a successful intermittent fast.

It is necessary to remember to keep your goals in your mind all the time. You may write them down somewhere. It will allow you to keep them in mind all the time.

Secondly, it is necessary to keep an eye on the strategy you are planning to follow. For instance, if you are planning to follow an alternate day fast continue with it until you start seeing results. When you stop seeing results, it is time to change your routine. If you find short fasts easier as compared to longer fasts, try alternating between them. You should also adjust your fast according to the seasons and atmosphere. For instance, less-frequent fasts are better in winters while shorter fasts are great in summers. Adapt and change. This will keep your body active and metabolism on its toes. Let us now have a look at the top fasting tips that will help you fast.

Fasting Tips:
Water is your friend

As said earlier, water is your best friend while fasting. Water is a non-caloric drink, i.e., it contains zero calories. It will keep your body hydrated. Dehydration is a common side effect associated with fasting and water will help you tackle it effectively. Water also has appetite-suppressing properties. Drink 2-3 cups of water every time you feel hungry, and it will make your feelings go away. It is always recommended to start your day with 2-3 cups of water. This will wake up your body, and you will feel hydrated throughout the day.

It is best to drink water in small sips. When water is drunk in small increments it combines with saliva and has the effect of neutralizing the acidity from the stomach and actually hydrates your body. Also, don't drink water 30 minutes before a meal.

Stay Active/Busy

One of the major reasons why people fail to fast is that they continuously think of food and eating. While it is understandable that a hungry mind will think of food, however, if you manage to keep your mind busy you will effectively stop thinking about food. While sedentary days are best for fasting, try doing it on a busy day. You will be too busy to think about hunger or food.

Coffee

After water, coffee is the best friend of fasters. Coffee is a mild appetite suppressant and 2-3 cups of coffee throughout the day will keep hunger at bay. Black coffee is the best way to drink coffee while fasting.

Tea

Tea is a great option for people who do not want to drink coffee. You can have a variety of teas while fasting. Do not add cream, milk or sugar to your tea. Green tea is one of the best options while fasting. Free tea contains chemicals that can suppress appetite. It also contains antioxidants that are great for your overall health.

Understand the Patterns of Hunger

Hunger does not work in a straight line; it comes and goes in waves. Hunger is not constant. Whenever you feel hungry, try to drink a cup of green tea or any other non-caloric beverage. This will keep you satiated.

Friends and Family

While friends and family can help you with communal fasting, they may hinder your progress in solo fasting. Many people will try to discourage you just because they do not understand the workings and benefits of fasting. While a close-knit group of friends and supporters can help you with your fast, a bunch of naysayers will harm you.

Nutritious diet

Intermittent fasting is a diet that promotes weight loss. If you want to lose weight, you should keep an eye on calories and diet. Many people think that intermittent fasting means eating anything they want when they are not fasting. It is not an excuse to eat whatever you like. While it is okay to indulge once in a while, you should continue to eat a low-carb, low-sugar and nutritious diet when you are not fasting. This will keep your body in the 'fat-burning' mode and will help you lose weight effectively.

One Month

Intermittent fasting is not a fad diet, and therefore it does not show instant results. You need to give it some time. You also need to give your body some time, as it will need some time to adjust to your new diet. Do not expect to lose weight in a couple of days, keep working towards your goal.

Lifestyle changes

Do not force a fast in your lifestyle, instead, try to adjust and find a fast that is compatible with your life. Do not change your life so that you can fast. This will only make you unhappy. Instead, try to fit your fast in your schedule in such a way that you will continue to enjoy your life while reaping the health benefits of intermittent fasting. If you want to celebrate holidays, do not force yourself to fast, instead enjoy and indulge (lightly). Once you are done with feasting, you can always compensate by fasting more. Remember, what makes fasting different than other diets is that it is flexible.

Avoid Binging

While overcompensating for fasts is a difficult task, it is not impossible. Try not to binge after fasting. Try to eat nutritious and healthy food only.

Breaking your fast

Once your fast is over, it is time to break it. Breaking fasts is a gradual process; you should not stuff yourself with a lot of food right after your fast. This is especially true in the case of longer fasts. The longer your fast was, the gentler your break must be. Many people tend to overeat right after the fast. This is not because they are hungry; rather it is due to the psychological need of eating. Overeating right after a fast may lead to stomach problems and discomfort.

When you want to break your fast, start slow with a small dish or a fruit. Wait for 30-60 minutes after which you can have your main meal. This 30-60 minute gap will allow the waves of hunger to pass, and you will not overeat.

Try to keep your pantry updated with healthy food items and veggies. While short-fasts require no special attention, fasts longer than a few hours do. It is always better to plan. You may keep your first snack ready in the refrigerator so that you can have your snack as soon as you plan to break your fast. Here's a list of things that can be your first snack after a long fast:

- One tablespoon almond butter and simple toast
- 1/4-cup almonds or any other nuts. (Not salted)
- A small bowl of salad
- A small bowl of raw veggies with vinegar and olive oil dressing.
- A small bowl of vegetable soup
- A small serving of plain meat.

While eggs can effectively be your first snack after a fast, it is recommended to avoid them. Many people feel abdominal distress after breaking fast with eggs. If you normally have a sensitive stomach, avoid eggs and eat fruit instead.

While breaking your fast, try to keep these things into your mind.

- Do not eat a lot of food and try to keep your serving sizes small. You will soon be eating a full meal anyway. If you stuff yourself with snacks first, you will feel bloated later.

- Chew thoroughly. Do not gorge and try to chew every bite carefully. Do not hurry. If you chew carefully, it will help your digestive system.

- Drink lots of water. Drink a tall glass of water before your snacks. People often forget or stop consuming fluids once their fast is over. This may lead to constipation and bloating. Try to keep yourself hydrated.

- Take your time. Do not hurry now that your fast is over. If you feel anxious about eating, try to keep calm.

Concerns

There are a few things that may concern you when you begin fasting. This section will try to cover some of these, one by one.

Hunger

Of course, the first and number one concern that people have about fasting is hunger. People assume that they will not be able to control their hunger that they will indulge in overeating. While most of the myths about hunger and fasting have already been addressed in the chapters above, let us have a look at some other myths associated with hunger.

Hunger, as explained above comes in waves, this means if you are feeling hungry at the moment, it will pass soon. You need to stay vigilant. Staying busy on the day of your fast will help you avoid hunger for a long time.

Once your body becomes accustomed to hunger, it will start burning the stores of fats. This will act as an appetite suppressor. After a week or two of regular fasting, you will stop feeling the pangs of hunger or your hunger will become less intense.

You can always drink water, green tea and other such beverages to help you tackle hunger. Along with the above drinks, there are a few spices and food items that can help you conquer hunger.

Cinnamon: Cinnamon is a great tasting, aromatic spice, and it also contains essential nutrients and chemicals that can help you suppress your hunger. It can help you lower your blood sugar level with ease. You can add cinnamon to your tea or coffee to make it tastier.

Chia Seeds: Chia seeds contain a lot of essential fiber and omega-3 fatty acids. These acids are good for the health of your heart. These seeds get absorbed easily in water and form a gel-like substance if they are soaked in water for more than 30 minutes. This gel can be eaten to satisfy your hunger. You can also eat these seeds dry. While eating chia seeds technically breaks the fast, it will help you to follow your fast more diligently.

Dizziness or Weakness

Another problem that people are worried about before starting a fast is dizziness. People believe that fasting may make them dizzy. This is half true.

Only misguided and unplanned fasting may cause weakness and dizziness. If you consume enough water and salt while fasting, you will not get dizzy. If you ever feel weak while fasting, have some homemade bone broth and you will feel good almost instantly.

Headaches

Headaches are a side effect of fasting, and almost all fasters will feel it at least once in their life. Headaches are especially common when you fast for the first couple of times. Don't worry. These headaches are common and temporary. Once your mind and body become accustomed to fasting, you will stop getting these headaches. Meanwhile, you may have some salt water or mineral water to control the headaches.

Constipation

Constipation or fewer bowel movements is a known side effect of fasting. When you fast your bowel movements will generally decrease, however, there is no need to worry, as it is the result of consuming less food. If you do not feel any discomfort or problem, there is no need to be anxious about decreased bowel movements. However, if you feel pain or trouble in emptying your bowels, you are not getting enough fiber. To counter this, eat Metamucil at least once a day. You can also incorporate oats into your diet.

Heartburn

Heartburn is another commonly associated problem with fasting. To avoid heartburn, do not consume a large meal right after you break your fast. Do not lie down immediately after eating and try to sit or stay in an upright position for some time after your meal. You can try drinking lemon with sparkling water. If the problem persists, contact a doctor.

Muscle Cramps

Muscle cramps are often caused due to deficiency of magnesium. While fasting it is possible that you may not get enough magnesium from your diet, in such cases, it is necessary to consume supplements. There are a lot of OTC magnesium supplements available on the market. If you do not want to take supplements, you can also try soaking in Epsom Salt. Make a warm bath and add 1 cup of Epsom salt to the tub. Soak in the bath for half an hour. Your body will absorb magnesium from your skin. You can also apply magnesium oil topically, and your skin will soak up the magnesium.

FAQs until now we saw some concerns and tips that will make your fasting experience worthwhile. In this section let us have a look at certain frequently asked questions.

Does fasting cause crankiness?

This phenomenon has not been observed in a lot of followers. It is assumed that fasting does not make you cranky. The only people who get cranky due to fasting are the people who believe that they will feel cranky. If you think optimistically you will not feel cranky at all. Instead of feeling cranky you will feel happy, refreshed and elated.

Will fasting make me weak or tired?

The simple answer to this question is no, fasting will not make you tired. Many people have reported feeling energized and elated while and after fasting. This goes completely against the myth that fasting will make you tired. Once you get accustomed to fasting, you will see that you now feel far more energized than regularly. A word of caution, if you feel excessively tired after or while fasting, stop fasting immediately and talk to a doctor as soon as possible.

Does fasting affect your memory negatively? OR Will fasting make me forgetful?

This is another relatively common concern. Fasting does not affect your memory or negatively retaining power. Rather it may cause positive changes in your mind and body. According to a popular theory, fasting causes autophagy, which means cellular cleansing. This cellular cleansing may help with memory loss and other age-related problems.

Will fasting make me overeat?

The simple answer to this question is yes. If you look at this question closely, you will realize that while fasting may cause overeating, it will not make you consume more calories than regular days. While people may consume larger meals after fasting, the net deficit of calories including the time of fasting and eating will still be negative. This means that you will still end up losing weight. It is difficult to compensate for fast, even if you overeat.

My stomach keeps growling and making weird noises while fasting. Is this common? What should I do?

This is a common phenomenon. When your stomach is empty, it makes sounds due to abdominal movements. You can stop this growling by drinking green tea or mineral water.

If you feel that your stomach is making too much noise, try drinking warm water mixed with a pinch of salt and a dash of lemon juice. After 30 minutes, make the same drink except with cold water this time. You can also add cinnamon and crushed black peppercorns to the above drink.

Can I do intermittent fast if I am on medications?

Yes, you can; however, you need to consult your doctor first. Certain medicines cannot be taken on an empty stomach as they may cause side effects. These medicines cannot be taken when you are fasting. Your doctor may recommend you to have a small meal to take medicine. Alternatively, you may adjust your fast according to your medicine schedule.

Can I fast if I have diabetes?

Yes, you can fast if you have diabetes, as fasting can help you with your blood sugar level. However, as diabetes is a high-risk disorder, it is necessary to contact your doctor before going on a fast. Do not modify your diet until contacting your doctor. You must monitor your blood sugar level and your health while fasting.

Can exercise and fasting go hand in hand?

Yes, you should incorporate some exercise into your daily schedule while fasting. This will increase the rate of weight loss and will also keep you energized. Exercise will also take your mind off food and hunger.

If you are an endurance trainer or athlete, it is recommended to contact your physician before starting a fast. Endurance training requires a lot of energy. These athletes often need to take supplements to fulfill this need for energy. Fasting may cause problems with their training. Therefore, always contact a health professional before starting a fast.

Chapter Twelve
How to Turn Intermittent Fasting Into a Healthy Habit?

Intermittent fasting is a beneficial and healthy diet plan, but following it can prove to be quite tricky. With some initial discipline, you can convert intermittent fasting into a habit, and with time your fasting experience will become effortless. Here are a few tips that will help you to turn intermittent fasting into a habit.

Thirty Days

According to science, it takes only 22 days to turn something into a habit while the initial stage may seem complicated, with enough practice and vigilance you will be able to condition your body and mind to get accustomed to intermittent fasting.

Start Simple

While 24-hour and 16/8 fast seem exciting, but they are difficult to pull off. It is recommended to go easy on your mind and body and start slow. Start with a short fast, which you can then extend gradually.

Reminders

We tend to forget things that we want to avoid. While fasting is beneficial, it is still something that people want to avoid. To help you form a habit of fasting, you can place reminders around your workplace or places that you see all the time. For instance, you may put cute reminders of your refrigerator, etc. You can also set reminders on your phone to remind you of your fast from time to time.

Get a friend

Peer pressure and peer support are both quite strong if you find fasting on your own difficult, rope in a friend to fast with you. Your friend will keep you motivated and vice versa.

Get rid of Temptation

It is difficult to control our tongue especially if you keep on seeing delicious food items all around you. If you live alone, get rid of all snacks and other unhealthy items and instead fill your pantry with healthy food items.

Stock up healthy items

The idea is to eat healthy and nutritious food in your feasting window too. Ensure your pantry is stocked with fresh fruit, vegetables and lean proteins. Refer to chapter 7 for a list of things you should consume.

If you manage to do all of the above things consistently, before you know it, you will be able to make intermittent fasting a way of life, which will improve your overall wellbeing and also help you maintain weight.

Conclusion

Thank you once again for buying this book, and I hope you found it interesting, informative and entertaining. I hope you will start to notice positive changes in your life after reading this.

As explained, Intermittent fasting is a not a fad diet rather it is a lifestyle choice. It is a great option for everyone who wants to lose weight, burn fat, look fit and get into better shape. Remember, diet is not just about the foods that you eat. It is also about the time you eat them. This is the basic principle of intermittent fasting. Try to understand your hunger and time your fasts accordingly, and you will start losing weight without any trouble.

What makes intermittent fasting difficult is that we often do not have self-control. People with extremely low self-control will find this diet difficult as compared to others. We have been taught that eating at least six meals a day is necessary for a healthy body and an active mind. While you may consume six, or even more meals throughout the day, these meals need to be small. Not many people can control their portions, which ultimately leads to drastic results. In intermittent fasting, you don't have to work hard like other diets to see positive results.

Remember, intermittent fasting is not just a fad diet; it tries to change your life for good. It has a multitude of benefits. Therefore, this diet will not only make you slim, but it will also help you become healthier and disease free.

This book has started your journey towards health and fitness. It is now in your hands to take the next step and go that extra mile to achieve your ideal body. Whether you are trying to lose weight or keep your diabetes under control, intermittent fasting can help you with everything- if you are ready to work hard.

This book contains all that is to know about intermittent fasting right from the type of intermittent fasts, diet plans, benefits of intermittent fasting and problems and risks of intermittent fasting as well. This book has tried to focus as much as possible on the scientific aspect of intermittent fasting making it highly informative. You can use this information to bring in positive changes in your life.

So don't wait, start fasting today!

Reference

https://www.health.harvard.edu/blog/intermittent-fasting-surprising-update-2018062914156

https://idmprogram.com/fasting-a-history-part-i/

https://www.dietdoctor.com/intermittent-fasting

https://www.bbc.com/news/health-44005092

https://idmprogram.com/difference-calorie-restriction-fasting-fasting-27/

https://www.mindbodygreen.com/articles/is-intermittent-fasting-really-good-for-women

https://www.ncbi.nlm.nih.gov/pmc/articles/PMC4508256/

https://www.ncbi.nlm.nih.gov/pubmed/28735644

https://www.dummies.com/health/nutrition/weight-loss/who-should-and-shouldnt-fast/

https://www.marksdailyapple.com/who-should-and-shouldnt-try-fasting/

https://www.medicalnewstoday.com/articles/319394.php

https://www.ncbi.nlm.nih.gov/pmc/articles/PMC3680567

https://www.healthline.com/nutrition/10-health-benefits-of-intermittent-fasting#section3

https://www.healthline.com/nutrition/10-health-benefits-of-intermittent-fasting#section3

https://www.businessinsider.com/benefits-of-intermittent-fasting-disease-fighting-weight-loss-2018-3#several-studies-suggest-that-intermittent-fasting-can-do-more-than-help-people-lose-weight-it-also-may-improve-blood-pressure-and-help-the-body-process-fat-1

https://www.businessinsider.com/benefits-of-intermittent-fasting-disease-fighting-weight-loss-2018-3#there-may-be-evolutionary-reasons-why-depriving-ourselves-of-food-for-some-time-makes-us-feel-energetic-and-focused-3

https://www.google.com/search?client=firefox-b-ab&q=what+is+startvation+mode

https://www.thisisinsider.com/intermittent-fasting-myths-2018-8

https://medium.com/@drstephanie/want-to-burn-fat-without-ever-stepping-foot-into-a-gym-think-fast-eac5c2a5d203

https://www.healthline.com/nutrition/11-myths-fasting-and-meal-frequency

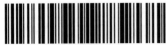

Made in the USA
Middletown, DE
04 July 2019